Your Health Your Power

A Healthcare Navigation Guide for Men Who Have Sex with Men

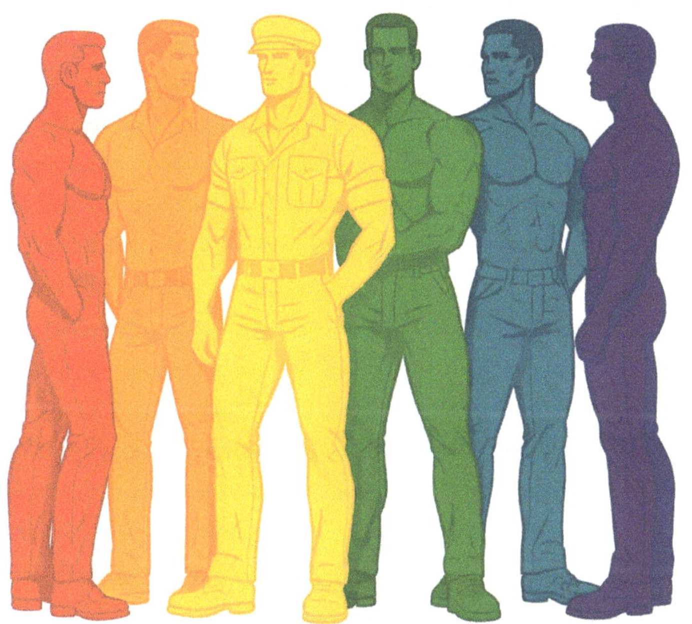

Dr Thomas Jude

Dr. Thomas Jude

Your Health, Your Power:
A Healthcare Navigation Guidebook for Men Who Have Sex with Men

Your Health, Your Power: A Healthcare Navigation Guide for Men Who Have Sex With Men

Dr. Thomas Jude

Cover Design by Tom of P-Town
ISBN: 979-8-218-83211-7
Library of Congress Control Number: 2025922219
Printed in the United States of America
Published in Provincetown, MA

Dedication

To Auntie Monnie —

Who opened her door and her heart when the world felt unsafe;
who taught me that intelligence means service;
who loved me into believing I could be more.

Your refuge became my foundation,
your lessons my compass,
your faith my wings.

This book exists because you saved my life
and showed me how to thrive.

With boundless gratitude and love,

Tommy

Foreword by Carolyn Savini MSN

As a fellow clinician, I have long admired colleagues who bridge the gap between science and humanity. Medicine, at its best, is not only about diagnosing disease or prescribing treatment it's about listening, affirming, and building trust. Few embody this better than Dr. Tom.

For decades, Dr. Tom has been both a healer and an advocate for men who have sex with men (MSM). His work has been shaped not only by deep expertise in HIV medicine, but by lived experience loss, resilience, and an unwavering commitment to ensuring that healthcare sees and serves our communities fully. In every lecture he gives, every clinic visit he conducts, and now in this book, he reminds us that health is not simply about survival but also about thriving.

This patient companion is an extraordinary achievement. It takes the rigor of medical science and translates it into clear, direct, and affirming guidance. Here, readers will find practical roadmaps on HIV prevention and treatment, STI screening, mental health, harm reduction, and more. But beyond the information, what strikes me most is the tone: respectful, unflinching, and empowering. Too often, patients have been left to navigate healthcare with shame or silence. This book insists on a different future one where questions are welcomed, bodies are respected, and care is tailored to real lives.

As clinicians, we know that our patients do best when they feel heard, understood, and supported. This companion doesn't replace the provider–patient relationship it strengthens it. By equipping readers with knowledge and confidence, it sets the stage for deeper collaboration in the exam room and beyond.

Dr. Thomas Jude

I believe this work will not only educate but also heal. It carries within it the spirit of solidarity and the hard-won belief that every gay, bi, and queer man deserves competent, compassionate, and affirming care. Dr. Tom has given us more than a book; he has given us a blueprint for better health and a reminder of what medicine, at its heart, is meant to be.

Caroyn Savini, MSN FNP

Disclaimer

This book is intended as an **informational resource** and **framework to facilitate discussion** between patients and their licensed medical providers. It is **not a substitute for professional medical advice, diagnosis, or treatment.**

Every person's health situation is unique. The information in this book is designed to **help you be informed and empowered** when talking with your healthcare provider about your care. You should never disregard or delay seeking professional medical advice because of something you read here.

If you have a medical emergency, call **911** or go to the nearest emergency department immediately.

This book is written to support open, honest, and informed conversations. If you feel that your current provider is unfamiliar with the specific health needs of men who have sex with men (MSM), you may wish to share with them our companion textbook, ***Primary Care of Men Who Have Sex with Men***, which was created as a resource for healthcare professionals.

Your health deserves care that is respectful, knowledgeable, and affirming. Use the information in these pages as a tool to ask questions, advocate for yourself, and build a collaborative partnership with your provider.

Preface to the Patient Companion

Healthcare hasn't always been kind—or even competent—when it comes to gay, bi, and queer men. Too many of us have walked into exam rooms only to feel judged, misunderstood, or outright ignored. The result? Higher rates of HIV and hepatitis, more struggles with mental health and substance use, and a lingering mistrust of a system that should have our backs.

I'm **Dr. Tom**—an HIV specialist, and, most importantly, a fellow member of this community. Long before I wore a white coat, I worked in virology labs hunting for better HIV treatments. Then, in 1996, I lost my partner to AIDS. That loss changed everything: I went back to school, became a clinician, and promised myself I would spend the rest of my career making healthcare safer, smarter, and kinder for men who have sex with men.

Over the past two decades I've cared for hundreds of guys—city kids and small-town transplants, leather daddies and circuit bros, monogamous partners and polycules—all looking for the same thing: a provider who listens and a plan that works. This book is my way of putting what I've learned into your hands.

What you'll find inside

- **Straight talk about sex and health.** Whether it's PrEP, PEP, lube choices, or kink safety, you deserve facts without blushes or judgment.
- **Practical roadmaps.** Vaccination schedules, STI testing timelines, mental-health check-ins, harm-reduction tips, and checklists to bring to your next appointment.

- **Tools for self-advocacy.** How to spot red flags in a clinic, push back against myths, and find LGBTQ+-affirming care—even if you live miles from the nearest gay-friendly neighborhood.
- **Hope.** Because we've come a long way, and with the right information and support, thriving is the expectation, not the exception.

This companion isn't just a spin-off of my provider facing textbook "Primary Care of Men Who Have Sex with Men"; it's a conversation between us. I've woven in the science, yes, but also the stories and strategies that have kept my patients—and myself—healthy, proud, and very much alive.

To the friends I've lost, the patients who continue to teach me, and every reader who's ever wondered if a doctor's office could feel like home: this book is for you. Let's make your next chapter one of power, knowledge, and unapologetic health. Special thanks to Tom Brennan, Tommy Wiles, and Kristyn Gonzalez.

With gratitude and solidarity,

Dr. Tom

Patient Companion — Table of Contents

Appendices & Quick-Grab Resources

Chapter 1

Why This Book Exists — Why Competent Care Matters for Gay, Bi & Queer Men

I want to start with a story about a friend of mine. He's smart, educated, and confident about who he is as a gay man. He has a primary care provider who is straight, but not at all homophobic—actually, quite the opposite. His doctor was open, supportive, and even willing to prescribe PrEP when my friend asked for it. He also made sure to include routine STI testing at my friend's PrEP check-ins. On the surface, this looks like a success story: a patient who feels comfortable, and a doctor who listens.

But here's the problem. This doctor only knew how to screen for gonorrhea and chlamydia by checking urine. He didn't know that gonorrhea and chlamydia can also infect the throat and the rectum, and that swabs of those areas are the only way to detect those infections when there. He wasn't being dismissive—he just wasn't trained to think about it. So for years, my friend—who thought he was being "screened for everything"—had never once had an anal or oral STI test.

This is such a simple example, but it shows the gap perfectly. Both the patient and the provider wanted to do the right thing. They had good communication. The doctor wasn't biased or homophobic. And yet, the care was incomplete and potentially unsafe. Why? Because LGBTQ+ health isn't part of the standard medical training most providers receive.

That's exactly why this companion exists. Our textbook "Primary Care of Men Who Have Sex with Men" can give providers the science and the tools to deliver competent care but they don't all know about or have it. Which brings us to this book—your book—it's here for you, the patient, so you can understand what care you should be getting, know to ask the right questions, and make sure nothing important gets missed in the case your provider just doesn't know. Because wanting to do the right thing isn't always enough—you need knowledge too.

1. From "Mental Disorder" to Medical After-Thought

Fifty-plus years ago, simply loving another man could earn you a psychiatric diagnosis. Homosexuality remained in the *Diagnostic and Statistical Manual of Mental Disorders* until 1973, when activists and allied clinicians finally forced the American Psychiatric Association to vote it out.

That victory ended official pathologizing, but it did **not** insert LGBTQ+ health into medical curricula. The legacy is still felt every time a provider blushes at the word "bottoming," skips an anal Pap test, or assumes "you must be married to a woman."

2. The Numbers That Prove the System Still Falls Short

Health Issue	What the Data Show	Why It Signals a Competency Gap

Health Issue	What the Data Show	Why It Signals a Competency Gap
HIV	Gay and bisexual men made up **67 %** (25,482) of all new U.S. HIV diagnoses in 2022.	Prevention (PrEP, PEP) and early treatment hinge on providers who understand modern HIV care.
Syphilis	MSM accounted for **32.7 %** of all primary & secondary syphilis cases in 2023—**57.5 %** of the cases among men.	Rising syphilis means clinicians must know how to look for and recognize primary and secondary cases and offer same-day treatment.
Missed STI Testing	Only **57.5 %** of U.S. clinics offer routine throat/rectal (extragenital) chlamydia + gonorrhea tests; ¾ of those clinics do it **only if the patient asks**.	When clinicians don't test where the infections actually live, diagnoses are missed and partners stay at risk.

Health Issue	What the Data Show	Why It Signals a Competency Gap
Hidden Infections	Community surveys show **1 in 8** MSM had an asymptomatic rectal or throat infection in a single screening round.	Routine, correct-site screening prevents silent spread and complications.
Anal Cancer	MSM who are HIV-negative are ~20× more likely to develop anal cancer than the general population; HIV-positive MSM face ~40× the risk.	Few clinicians outside LGBTQ+ clinics discuss anal-Pap or high-resolution anoscopy.
Mental Health	In 2023, **26 %** of LGB high-school students attempted suicide—five times the rate of straight peers.	Affirming care and early mental-health referral literally save lives.

Bottom line: The disparities are not "just how it is." They are the measurable fallout of training gaps, stigma, and rushed visits where essential questions go unasked.

3. Why an *Informed* Provider Changes Everything

- A provider who knows that rectal gonorrhea is often silent will swab, not shrug.

- A provider who understands gay sexual networks will talk PrEP *and* U=U, not either/or.
- A provider comfortable discussing chemsex, steroid cycles, or pup play can offer harm-reduction instead of moral lectures.

When competence meets cultural humility, the statistics above begin to shift—toward earlier diagnoses, fewer infections, and stronger mental-health outcomes.

4. Your Turn — Mapping What Makes *Your* Health Unique

Grab a notebook or open your phone. Reflect honestly; no one sees this but you.

Prompt	Check Your Box
Sexual Practices — Do you engage in receptive anal sex, group sex, kink/fetish play (e.g., fisting, sounding, breath control)?	□ Yes □ No
STI Risk — How often are you screened at *all* sites (throat, rectum, urine/penis)?	□ Quarterly □ Yearly □ Rarely
Substances — Any use of party drugs (meth, GHB, poppers, cocaine) or chemsex patterns?	□ Yes □ No

Prompt	Check Your Box
Performance & Image — Have you used anabolic steroids, peptide hormones, or high-dose supplements?	□ Yes □ No
Mental Health — Recent feelings of persistent sadness, anxiety, or thoughts of self-harm?	□ Yes □ No
Vaccines — Up to date on HPV, meningococcal (ACWY + B), hepatitis A/B, Mpox?	□ All □ Some □ Unsure

Exercise Goal: Circle any "Yes," "Rarely," or "Unsure." Each one points to a topic that benefits from an LGBTQ-competent clinician in your corner. Keep this list; you'll use it in the next chapter when we talk about *how* to find that provider.

Key Takeaways

- Queer health disparities trace back to history, stigma, and under-training—not biology.
- Hard numbers on HIV, syphilis, anal cancer, and mental health make a watertight case for culturally competent care.
- Identifying your own risk landscape prepares you to advocate for the screenings, vaccinations, and conversations you deserve.

Chapter 2

Finding Affirming Care & Overcoming Medical Mistrust

Opening story: why affirming care isn't "nice to have"—it's essential

Picture me an educated provider, clutching an MRI disc like a golden ticket—the very test that *does* help diagnose ano-rectal fistulas—walking into a big-deal Boston hospital feeling hopeful. The surgeon barely glanced at me, never looked at the disc, and confidently announced, "MRIs can't diagnose fistulas." (They can and in fact are the gold-standard). He then did an exam, called me "a homosexual" more than once, told me I had anal warts (I didn't—I had an ano-rectal fistula and a hemorrhoid), and, as a final flourish, left an instrument in my underwear that literally fell out while I was walking down the hall after. Not exactly the "world-class" vibe I was going for.

I left feeling embarrassed, angry, and honestly a little heartsick. I'm a clinician, and *even I* hesitated to report it because reliving the appointment felt exhausting. If you've ever swallowed a bad healthcare experience just to avoid more stress—you're not alone.

A week later, I saw an LGBTQ-affirming colorectal surgeon at another major center. She popped the MRI disc into a computer, calmly confirmed the fistula, and walked me through both surgical and conservative options like a partner, not a problem. She also took care of the hemorrhoid and verified I did not have any anal warts. When I told her about the prior visit, she gently said what I needed to hear: "You should have reported him." She was right. Because what happened to me isn't some rare oddity—too many LGBTQ+

folks experience care that's dismissive, biased, or just plain wrong.

Here's the point: finding affirming, evidence-based care isn't about being picky—it's about getting safe, accurate, respectful medicine. When someone refuses to review your records, misnames you, fixates on your identity, or makes you feel small, that's not "bedside manner." That's a red flag.

This chapter is your roadmap to avoiding the red flags and finding the green ones: how to vet clinics, what to say on the phone before you book, how to bring a buddy or an advocate, scripts for shutting down bias in the moment, and what to do if you're dismissed or disrespected (including how to report it—*if you have the bandwidth*). **You deserve care that treats your body** and **your dignity like they both matter—because they do.**

1. Why Trust Feels Risky—And Why It's Worth Re-Building

Just like my story many gay, bi, and queer men carry medical "battle scars." Studies show LGBTQ+ adults report **higher rates of medical gaslighting, trauma, and outright distrust** than their straight peers. That mistrust makes perfect sense—history taught us caution. But when fear keeps you away from clinics, silent infections stay silent, mental-health symptoms smolder, and small problems snowball. Re-learning to trust the *right* clinicians is therefore a critical health skill, not a luxury.

2. What Affirming Care Looks (and Feels) Like

Green-Flag Behaviors	Red-Flag Behaviors
Intake forms include your pronouns and avoid "married / single" only	Forms force "husband / wife," no space for partners or sexual orientation
Staff use partners' names without smirking or surprise	Staff whisper or exchange looks when you mention a same-sex partner
Provider initiates conversations about sexual practices, PrEP, Doxy-PEP, vaccines	You must bring up every LGBTQ-specific topic yourself
Three-site STI screening offered as routine care	Only urine sample taken, no throat or rectal testing despite risk factors
Clear referrals to LGBTQ-affirming therapists, surgeons, recovery programs	"I don't know anyone who does that" or "Just Google it"

When green flags outnumber red flags, you've probably found a solid match—one that will protect against the diagnostic misses and stigma-driven delays described in Chapter 1.

3. Where to Start the Search

Resource	Why It's Useful
OutList® (OutCareHealth.org) – 10,000+ affirming providers searchable by zip code	Lets you filter by specialty, insurance, telehealth; free
GLMA / LGBTQ+ Healthcare Directory – National database relaunched in 2022	Especially strong for primary care & mental health providers glma.orgLGBTQ+ Healthcare Directory
Telehealth PrEP & STI Platforms (e.g., Folx, Mistr)	Secure online consults, at-home labs, meds shipped discreetly—handy if local options are scarce MISTR
Local LGBTQ Centers, AIDS Service Orgs	Often keep vetted referral lists and know who's culturally competent in your area
Planned Parenthood / FQHCs	Sliding-scale fees, increasingly train staff in LGBTQ-inclusive care

4. Screening a Potential Provider—Five Quick Questions

Call or send a portal message before booking:

1. **"Does the practice prescribe and manage PrEP and Doxy-PEP?"**

2. **"How often do you perform throat and rectal swabs for STI screening in MSM?"** (Missed extragenital testing hides ~13 % of infections.PMC)
3. **"Are your staff trained in LGBTQ cultural humility?"**
4. **"Do you offer or refer for anal-Pap or high-resolution anoscopy when indicated?"**
5. **"Do intake forms allow patients to list pronouns and chosen names?"**

A confident, informed "Yes" (or a thoughtful explanation) to most questions signals readiness. Hesitation or ignorance? Keep looking.

5. Preparing for the First Appointment

- **Pack a One-Page Health Snapshot** – Current meds, allergies, past STIs, vaccines, mental-health history, substance use.
- **Bring Your Risk Map** – The checklist you completed in Chapter 1 helps focus the visit.
- **Decide Your Deal-Breakers** – If a provider dismisses condomless receptive sex as "low risk," or seems shocked by chemsex, you're free to exit.
- **Know Your Rights** – Discrimination based on sexual orientation or gender identity violates Section 1557 of the Affordable Care Act; many states add extra protections.

6. Healing Medical Mistrust

1. **Start Small** – Book a PrEP refill or vaccine visit; gauge the vibe before entrusting deeper issues.
2. **Use Written Communication** – Patient portals let you clarify doubts without face-to-face anxiety.
3. **Bring an Ally** – A trusted friend can take notes and provide backup if conversations get tense.
4. **Give Feedback (Safely)** – Many clinics welcome anonymous surveys; constructive notes can improve care for the next guy.
5. **Switch If Needed—Guilt-Free** – You owe loyalty to your health, not to a disappointing provider.

7. Exercise—Your Personal Care-Hunt Blueprint

Task	Target Date	Done?
Identify **three** potential providers/directories to explore	___ / ___ / 20__	☐
Call or message each with the **five screening questions**	___ / ___ / 20__	☐
Compare answers; shortlist one provider for a first visit	___ / ___ / 20__	☐
Draft or update your **One-Page Health Snapshot**	___ / ___ / 20__	☐
Schedule initial appointment (in-person or telehealth)	___ / ___ / 20__	☐

Tackle the checklist at your own pace; every box you tick chips away at mistrust and moves you toward care you can trust.

Key Takeaways

- **Affirming care is identifiable**—green flags outshine red when you know what to look for.
- **Directories and telehealth** expand options far beyond your immediate ZIP code.
- **Preparation + screening questions** transform you from a passive patient into an empowered client.
- **Re-building trust** is a process; small positive encounters lay the groundwork for long-term health partnerships.

Chapter 3

Your Preventive Toolkit – Check-Ups, Screenings, and The Vaccines That Matter

When it comes to vaccines, the headlines these days can be confusing—and sometimes downright misleading. If you spend even a little time online, you'll find people arguing about whether vaccines are "safe," often with more passion than evidence. As of August 2025, let me be crystal clear: every vaccine currently approved and recommended for gay men by the FDA is incredibly safe. The science is solid, the benefits are enormous, and the risks are minimal.

I don't say this lightly. Over the years, I've cared for patients who developed oral cancers caused by HPV. These are not abstract risks—they're devastating realities. I've seen people endure brutal surgeries that removed parts of their tongues, jaws, and throats. These procedures save lives, but they're invasive, disfiguring, and agonizing. And the truth is, many of these cancers are preventable. That's why the HPV vaccine in particular feels like one of the greatest scientific achievements of our time.

When the HPV vaccine first came out, it was only recommended for younger people. I was technically "too old" to get it under the guidelines. But I knew the science, and I knew it would likely work for me. So, I pulled out my credit card and paid nearly a thousand dollars to complete the series out of pocket. A lot of money, yes, but worth every penny. Not long after, the recommendation age was raised to 45, proving my suspicion right. To this day, I consider it one of the best investments I've ever made in my own health.

This chapter is about building your prevention toolkit—vaccines, screenings, and other strategies that protect you before problems start. In the world of men's health, especially gay men's health, prevention is not just smart. It's life-changing.

Why Bother With Prevention?

Many gay, bisexual, and queer men grew up thinking of health care as something you seek **after** something feels wrong. Preventive care turns that idea on its head. By checking in regularly, you can:

- Catch silent problems early, when they are easiest to treat.
- Avoid long-term complications that can shorten or limit your life.
- Build a steady, respectful partnership with a clinician who understands your specific health needs.

Because certain infections and cancers appear more often—or in slightly different ways—in men who have sex with men, an ordinary "one-size-fits-all" checklist is not enough. The pages that follow give you a clear, step-by-step plan you can bring to every appointment.

The Building Blocks of Routine Care

Building Block	What Happens	How Often (Typical)
Yearly Comprehensive Visit	A head-to-toe physical exam, discussion of mental health, lifestyle review, blood work, and updating vaccines.	Every **twelve months**.
Problem-Focused Visits	Follow-up of ongoing issues such as high blood pressure, diabetes, or human immunodeficiency virus management.	As recommended by your clinician.
Telehealth or Same-Day Visits	Brief video or phone appointments for new symptoms, prescription refills, or quick sexually transmitted infection testing after a potential exposure.	Any time a new concern comes up.

Tip: If you have risk factors—such as living with human immunodeficiency virus, taking gender-affirming hormones, or using certain recreational drugs—your clinician may suggest more frequent check-ups.

When you book tests, do not be shy about asking for them by name and understanding what each one does. Below is a plain-language guide.

Test Name & What It Checks	Why You Might Need It	How Often to Ask For It
Comprehensive Sexually Transmitted Infection Panel • *Human Immunodeficiency Virus Antibody/Antigen Blood Test* • *Syphilis Treponemal Antibody Blood Test* • *Urine Test for Chlamydia and Gonorrhea* • *Throat Swab for Chlamydia and Gonorrhea* • *Rectal Swab for Chlamydia and Gonorrhea*	Sexually transmitted infections often cause **no symptoms**. Extra-genital sites (throat and rectum) are common hiding places in men who have receptive oral or anal sex.	**Every three months** if you are sexually active with more than one partner, share toys, or share drug-use equipment. If you are in a mutually monogamous relationship and neither partner has other risks, every twelve months may be enough—discuss with your clinician.
Hepatitis B Surface Antigen Blood Test	Tells whether you have an ongoing (chronic) Hepatitis B infection. Chronic infection can slowly damage the liver.	Test once. Repeat only if you were not immune when first tested and you have new risk factors, such as sharing drug

Test Name & What It Checks	Why You Might Need It	How Often to Ask For It
		equipment, or unprotected sex.
Hepatitis C Antibody Blood Test	Detects current or past Hepatitis C infection, which can also harm the liver.	At least once. Repeat **every year** if you share injection or intranasal drug equipment, get new tattoos or piercings, or share sex toys.
Anal Cancer Screening (Anal Pap Smear or High-Resolution Anoscopy)	Human papillomavirus (the wart virus) can lead to anal cancer, especially in people living with human immunodeficiency virus or anyone who regularly receives anal sex or uses anal toys.	**Every one to two years** if any of the risk factors apply.

Test Name & What It Checks	Why You Might Need It	How Often to Ask For It
Colon Cancer Screening (Stool Test or Colonoscopy)	Looks for early polyps or cancers in the large intestine.	Starting at age forty-five. A yearly stool test called "fecal immunochemical test" is simple if average risk; a colonoscopy every three (high risk) to ten years is an alternative.
Prostate Cancer Screening (Prostate-Specific Antigen Blood Test and Possibly a Digital Rectal Exam)	Detects early prostate changes.	Start talking about it at age fifty (age forty-five if you are Black or have a family history). The decision is shared between you and your clinician.
Liver Ultrasound With Alpha-Fetoprotein Blood Test	Screens for liver cancer in people with chronic Hepatitis B or liver scarring (cirrhosis).	**Every six months** if you fall into those groups.

Test Name & What It Checks	Why You Might Need It	How Often to Ask For It
General Metabolic and Mental-Health Checks • Blood Pressure • Body Mass Index • Cholesterol Panel • Hemoglobin A1c (long-term blood-sugar level) • Depression and Anxiety Questionnaires • Substance-Use Screening	Heart disease, diabetes, mood disorders, and substance-use issues can creep up silently.	Blood pressure and weight: **each visit.** Cholesterol and Hemoglobin A1c: every three years starting at thirty-five (or yearly if you have risk factors). Mood and substance-use screens: at least once a year or whenever you notice changes.

Vaccines: What They Protect You From and Why They Matter

Vaccines are not just for childhood. Below are the shots most relevant for gay, bisexual, and queer men, explained in plain English. At the time of this publication the US is experiencing a resurgence of measles. You should ask your provider to check your antibody titer and if you do not have immunity an MMR booster should be added to your vaccine to-do list!

Foundational Vaccines (Everyone Should Have These)

Vaccine Name	How You Catch the Illness	What the Illness Looks Like	Why the Shot Is Important	When You Need It
Tetanus, Diphtheria, and Whooping Cough Vaccine	Tetanus enters through cuts; the other two spread in the air with coughing etc.	Tetanus causes severe muscle spasms; diphtheria blocks breathing; whooping cough is a violent, long-lasting cough and can be deadly for babies.	Protects you and prevents you from spreading to infants.	1 Adult dose, then a booster **every 10 years**. If you have contact with a newborn, you may need an extra booster.

Vaccine Name	How You Catch the Illness	What the Illness Looks Like	Why the Shot Is Important	When You Need It
Seasonal Influenza (Flu) Shot	Spread by droplets in the air.	High fever, aching muscles, sometimes pneumonia or inflammation of the heart.	Men living with HIV, smokers, and asthmatics are hit harder by the flu.	**Every autumn**, before flu season starts. People older than sixty-five get a high-dose version.
COVID-19 Vaccine	Spread by airborne particles.	Can range from a mild cold to severe pneumonia, blood clots, death and "long COVID."	People with immune compromise, excess weight, or heart disease are at higher risk of lasting problems.	Complete the initial series then get the **updated booster each fall** (follow current public-health guidance).

High-Priority Vaccines for Gay, Bisexual, and Queer Men

Vaccine Name	Why MSM	What the Illness Does	Vaccine Details
Hepatitis A Vaccine	Oral-anal contact ("rimming"), sharing drugs, and food-borne outbreaks in gay social scenes.	Several weeks of fever, nausea, and yellow skin; rarely causes sudden liver failure and possible death.	Two-shot series: one now, the second **six months** later . Protection lasts decades.

Vaccine Name	Why MSM	What the Illness Does	Vaccine Details
Hepatitis B Vaccine	Spread through sex, blood, shared toys, and drug equipment. Human immunodeficiency virus co-infection speeds up liver damage.	Chronic infection can lead to cirrhosis (liver scarring) and liver cancer.	Traditional schedule: three shots over six months. New option: two shots, one month apart.
Nine-Valent Human Papillomavirus Vaccine	The wart virus causes anal, penile, and throat cancers more often in men who have sex with men.	Warts, cellular changes, cancers years later.	If you start before your fifteenth birthday: two shots six months apart. If you start later: three shots over six months. Approved up to age forty-five; older adults can discuss off-label use.

Vaccine Name	Why MSM	What the Illness Does	Vaccine Details
Meningococcal Group A, C, W, and Y Vaccine	Outbreaks have been linked to crowded bars, sex parties, and Pride festivals.	Sudden meningitis (brain and spinal-cord infection) or bloodstream infection; can be fatal within hours.	Two initial doses eight weeks apart, then a **booster every five years** while you remain at risk.
Meningococcal Group B Vaccine	This strain is not covered by the A, C, W, Y shot and spreads in the same settings.	Can cause tissue damage so severe that amputations are needed.	Two-dose series at least one month apart *or* a three-dose series over six months, depending on the brand your clinician carries.
Mpox (Monkeypox) Vaccine	Close skin-to-skin or sexual contact and shared bedding.	Painful blisters, swollen lymph	Two doses four weeks apart. If outbreaks

Vaccine Name	Why MSM	What the Illness Does	Vaccine Details
		nodes, rectal pain, and long isolation while contagious.	return or you have a weakened immune system, a booster may be advised later.

Age- or Condition-Specific Vaccines

Vaccine	Who Needs It	What It Prevents	Schedule
Shingles Vaccine (Recombinant Zoster Vaccine)	Everyone age fifty or older; people nineteen or older with weakened immunity (for example, from human immunodeficiency virus).	Shingles: a painful rash that can leave long-lasting nerve pain.	Two doses, with the second two to six months after the first.
Pneumococcal Conjugate Vaccine (Twenty-Valent)	Everyone age sixty-five or older; adults of any age who smoke or	Pneumonia, meningitis, bloodstream infections	One dose gives long-

Vaccine	Who Needs It	What It Prevents	Schedul e
	have lung, heart, liver disease, or live with human immunodeficienc y virus.	caused by the pneumococcu s bacterium.	term coverage; no follow-up shot is needed for most people.
Chickenpox (Varicella) Vaccine	Adults who never had chickenpox and were never vaccinated.	Chickenpox can be severe in adults and later re-emerge as shingles.	Two doses four to eight weeks apart.

Planning Your Appointment: A Four-Step Checklist

1. **Write Down Your Sexual History**
    - How many partners you have had recently.
    - The kinds of sex you enjoy (oral, anal, use of toys).
    - Whether you share toys or drug-use equipment.
2. **Photograph Your Vaccine Card**
   Keep a picture on your phone and mark any missing or overdue shots.
3. **List Your Goals in Advance**
   Examples:
    - "I need my three-month sexually transmitted infection panel."

   - "I would like the nine-valent human papillomavirus vaccine."
   - "Please explain injectable pre-exposure prophylaxis."

4. **Ask About Cost Before The Needle**
   Hepatitis A and B, human papillomavirus, and mpox vaccines are free at most health departments and are fully covered by the Affordable Care Act when given by an in-network clinician.

Quick Self-Check

Question	Yes / No
Have you had all three sexually transmitted infection tests—urine, throat swab, and rectal swab—within the last three months?	☐ / ☐
Are you fully vaccinated against Hepatitis A, Hepatitis B, and Human Papillomavirus?	☐ / ☐
In the past year, have you talked with a clinician about pre-exposure prophylaxis (including injectable options), post-exposure prophylaxis, or doxycycline after sex (often called doxy-PEP)?	☐ / ☐
Do you know your most recent blood pressure, cholesterol level, and long-term blood-sugar result (Hemoglobin A1c)?	☐ / ☐
Are you up to date on cancer screenings such as anal Pap smear and colonoscopy?	☐ / ☐

Circle any "No" answers and bring this page (or a photo of it) to your next visit.

7 | Key Takeaways

- **Every three months**: a complete sexually transmitted infection screen is the norm for sexually active gay, bisexual, and queer men.
- Vaccines like Hepatitis A and B, Human Papillomavirus, meningococcal, and mpox are must-haves—not extras.
- Prevention is an investment. By staying on top of checks and shots, you protect your own health and the health of your partners and community.
- If your clinician seems uncomfortable discussing these topics, remember: you deserve respectful, knowledgeable care. Keep looking until you find it.

Chapter 4

HIV Basics: Testing, Treatment, and Living Undetectable

When I was a young gay man in the 1990s, HIV was the monster in the room. I was working as a virologist, trying to help create a vaccine, and at the same time, I was falling in love. His name was Michael—my real-life Prince Charming. He was gorgeous, funny, and HIV positive. In 1996, I lost him to AIDS.

What crushed me wasn't just losing him but witnessing how the medical system treated him along the way. To many doctors, Michael was just "a case," a bundle of infections. Sitting there beside him, I remember thinking: *this isn't how this should be.* That experience is what inspired me to go into healthcare and influenced my decision to become a nurse practitioner, not an MD. I had just been accepted to medical school in Boston at the time. It seemed at the time as though MD's didn't receive any education on humanism just human bodies. I wanted to practice medicine in a way that saw patients as people first, not just as problems to solve. I thought at the time the difference between the two professions was that MD programs spent more time training on science but I was already a biological scientist.

Fast forward to today, and the world looks completely different. HIV is no longer a death sentence. With early diagnosis and modern treatment, people living with HIV can live a normal lifespan. Even more remarkably, science has given us U=U—undetectable equals untransmittable. If someone is on treatment for some time and their viral load is undetectable, they cannot pass HIV to their sexual partners. Period. That's not just stigma-reducing, that's relationship-saving, life-affirming science.

But let me be honest—it still takes trust, courage, and conversation to get there and it requires a patient provider relationship that is a safe space for open communication. In my own practice today, I have several patients who identifies as straight, are married to women, and quietly have sex with men on the side. One of them is living with HIV, and his wife doesn't know. For him, U=U isn't just a slogan—it's what keeps his marriage intact and his wife safe, even though she has no idea of the risks around her. That's a complicated, very human reality. And it's why open, nonjudgmental care matters so much.

This is exactly why this book exists. HIV has changed so dramatically since the days when I lost Michael—but managing it well still depends on knowledge, compassion, and safe spaces to tell the truth. In this chapter, we'll cover the basics: testing, treatment, and what it means to live undetectable today.

HIV (Human Immunodeficiency Virus) is a virus that attacks the immune system, which is your body's defense system against infections. Without treatment, HIV slowly damages the immune system over years, leaving the body more open to illnesses and certain cancers.

Today, HIV is treatable. With early diagnosis and daily medicine, people living with HIV can stay healthy, have a normal life expectancy, and avoid passing the virus to others.

How HIV Is Spread – and How Likely Is It?

HIV is present in certain body fluids—blood, semen, pre-seminal fluid (pre-cum), vaginal fluids, rectal fluids, and breast milk. For the virus to spread, these fluids must get into another person's bloodstream. This usually happens through:

- Unprotected sex (anal or vaginal)
- Sharing needles or syringes
- From mother to baby during pregnancy, birth, or breastfeeding if not treated

It **cannot** be spread by hugging, kissing, sharing toilets, towels, dishes, or touching.

Sexual Transmission Risks

HIV Transmission Risk by Activity

(Risk per single exposure if the partner with HIV is not on treatment and has a detectable viral load)

Activity	Estimated Risk per Act	Risk Level
Receptive anal sex ("bottoming")	~1.38% (1 in 72)	● **High**
Insertive anal sex ("topping")	~0.11% (1 in 909)	□ **Medium**
Receptive vaginal sex	~0.08% (1 in 1,250)	□ **Medium**
Insertive vaginal sex	~0.04% (1 in 2,500)	□ **Low**
Sharing needles or syringes	~0.63% (1 in 159)	● **High**
Receiving oral sex	Negligible risk	□ **Low**
Giving oral sex	Very low; slightly higher if sores/bleeding gums present	□ **Low**

Activity	Estimated Risk per Act	Risk Level
Kissing, touching, sharing toilets/dishes	No risk	□ **No risk**

How to Use This Chart

- These numbers are **averages**—actual risk depends on viral load, presence of other sexually transmitted infections, condom use, and prevention medicines.
- If the person with HIV is on treatment and **undetectable**, the risk is **zero for sexual transmission**.
- Combining prevention tools (condoms, PrEP, and regular testing) reduces your risk even more.

Other Ways HIV Can Spread

- **Sharing needles or syringes** – about **0.63% per act** (1 in 159)
- **Blood transfusions** – In countries with modern blood screening, the risk is extremely low (less than 1 in 2 million donations).
- **Mother-to-child** – Without treatment, 15–45% of babies born to mothers with HIV will get it. With treatment during pregnancy, birth, and breastfeeding, the risk drops to below 1%.
- **Occupational exposure (needle stick in healthcare)** – about **0.23% per injury** (1 in 435).

Acute HIV Infection – The Early Stage

After someone gets HIV, there's often a short period when the virus multiplies very quickly. This is called **acute HIV infection**, and it usually happens **2 to 4 weeks after exposure**.

About half to two-thirds of people will notice symptoms, which can include:

- Fever
- Sore throat
- Swollen lymph nodes (neck, armpits, groin)
- Rash on the body or face
- Headache
- Muscle aches and joint pain
- Night sweats
- Mouth ulcers

These symptoms are often mistaken for the flu, strep throat, or mononucleosis ("mono"). They usually go away in 1–2 weeks even without treatment—but the virus remains in the body.

The Latent Period – When HIV is Quiet

After the early stage, HIV enters a **latent period**. You may feel completely healthy during this time, which can last for years. But the virus is still active, slowly damaging the immune system.

Without treatment, the immune system will eventually become too weak to fight off certain infections and cancers. This is when HIV can progress to AIDS (Acquired Immune Deficiency Syndrome). With modern treatment, almost no one in countries with good medical care should ever progress to AIDS.

Why Testing Is So Important

Because you can have HIV for years without symptoms, the only way to know your status is to get tested. Testing also allows you to start treatment early, which protects your health and prevents transmission to others.

When to test:

- At least once a year if you are sexually active
- Every 3–6 months if you have multiple partners, are part of a sexual network where HIV is common, or share injection equipment
- After a possible exposure (some tests detect HIV as early as 10 days, others take longer)

Types of HIV Tests

1. **Rapid tests** – Give results in 20–30 minutes from a finger stick or mouth swab.
2. **Lab-based antibody tests** – Detect antibodies your body makes in response to HIV; usually positive 3–12 weeks after exposure.
3. **Combination (antigen/antibody) tests** – Can detect the virus earlier, within 2–4 weeks after infection.

If your first test is positive, the lab will confirm it with a second, different test before making a diagnosis.

Treatment – What You Need to Know

Treatment for HIV is called **antiretroviral therapy**. Most people take one pill once a day; some can get an injection every month or two. The medicines stop the virus from multiplying, which protects the immune system and reduces inflammation in the body.

Benefits of early treatment:

- Keeps your immune system strong
- Lets you live a normal life span
- Prevents sexual transmission (if undetectable)
- Lowers risk of other health problems like heart disease

What "Undetectable" Means

When HIV treatment works well, the amount of virus in your blood (viral load) drops so low that it can't be found by standard tests. This is called **undetectable**.

Undetectable = Untransmittable (U=U)
If you're undetectable and stay on treatment, you **cannot** pass HIV to your sexual partners. This has been proven in large studies. You still have HIV, and if you stop treatment, the virus will come back—but staying undetectable keeps you healthy and stops transmission.

Living Well with HIV

With the right care:

- You can live as long as someone without HIV.
- You can have relationships and sex without passing HIV to partners if undetectable.
- You can have HIV-negative children.
- You can live a full, active life.

Take your medicine daily, keep your medical appointments, eat well, stay active, and look after your mental health.

Key Takeaways

- HIV can be spread in different ways, with receptive anal sex carrying the highest sexual risk.
- Early symptoms may look like the flu—don't ignore them if you've had a possible exposure.
- You can feel fine for years while HIV is damaging your immune system—testing is the only way to know.
- Treatment makes HIV manageable and prevents passing it to others.
- Being undetectable means you can live your life without fear of giving HIV to sexual partners.

Patient Exercise:

- Think about your sexual practices—do you know the relative risks?
- When was your last HIV test?

- If you have HIV, do you know your current viral load?
- If you're HIV-negative, do you know about prevention options like daily pills, injections, and condoms?

Chapter 5

PrEP, PEP & U=U: Real-World Strategies to Stay HIV-Negative or Undetectable

As we bring this book to publication in the fall of 2025, it's still shocking to me that there are primary care providers who don't know how—or simply aren't interested—in prescribing PrEP or PEP. That gap matters, because for patients, access to PrEP, PEP, and the knowledge of U=U can literally mean the difference between staying HIV-negative, staying undetectable or being at peace.

One of the goals of this book is to empower *you* as a patient. That means giving you the language, the questions, and the knowledge to help guide your provider—if they're willing to learn. It means helping you recognize what competent care looks like, and what red flags to watch out for if a provider isn't prepared to meet your needs.

I can tell you that in my own practice, I haven't had to give a new HIV diagnosis in a very long time. That's not luck—that's prevention, treatment, and science working the way they're supposed to. My hope is that this becomes the reality for all providers everywhere: that new diagnoses become rare, and HIV stops being something anyone needs to fear.

This chapter will walk you through the prevention and treatment tools available today: how to access and use PrEP, what to do if you need PEP, and why U=U changes everything about what it means to live with HIV.

HIV prevention and treatment have come a long way. Today, we have tools so effective that ending new HIV infections is possible—if people know about them and can access them.

Three of the most powerful tools are:

- **PrEP** – medicines taken before possible exposure to prevent HIV infection
- **PEP** – medicines taken after a possible exposure to prevent HIV infection
- **U=U** – the fact that people with HIV who get to and remain undetectable cannot pass the virus sexually

Used correctly, these can be life-changing—whether you're HIV-negative and want to stay that way, or HIV-positive and want to protect your partners.

PrEP – Pre-Exposure Prophylaxis

What it is:
PrEP means taking HIV medicine regularly before being exposed to HIV, so the virus can't take hold in your body.

Who should consider it:

- Gay, bisexual, and other men who have sex with men who have condomless anal sex
- People who have a partner with HIV who is not consistently undetectable
- People who share needles or other injection equipment
- Anyone with an STI in the last year at ongoing risk

Types of PrEP and How They're Taken

1. **Daily oral pills** – taken every day at the same time

    - *Tenofovir disoproxil fumarate with emtricitabine* (generic Truvada) – for all genders
        - **Dose:** 1 pill once daily
    - *Tenofovir alafenamide with emtricitabine* (Descovy) – for men and transgender women; not approved (at this time August 2025) for those having receptive vaginal sex
        - **Dose:** 1 pill once daily
2. **On-demand (2-1-1) PrEP** – for some men who have sex with men
    - Take **2 pills 2–24 hours before sex**, then **1 pill 24 hours later**, then **1 pill 48 hours after the first dose**
    - Not FDA-approved in the U.S. yet and not recommended for people with vaginal exposure
3. **Long-acting injectable PrEP** – *Cabotegravir* given every 2 months by a healthcare provider
    - **Dose:** Injection in the buttock muscle every 8 weeks
4. **Extra-long acting injectable PrEP -** *Lenacapavir*– given every 6 months by a healthcare provider
    - **Dose:** Injection under the skin (Abdomen or Thigh) twice a year after initial start-up

Possible Side Effects of PrEP

Most people tolerate PrEP well. Possible side effects (Depending on which option you choose) include (your provider can give you specific side effects when starting you on one of the options):

- Nausea, diarrhea, or stomach upset (usually temporary)
- Headache

- Small decreases in kidney function (rare, usually reversible)
- Bone density changes (more with Truvada; mild and reversible)
- Injection site soreness, injection site reaction including infections for injectable PrEP

How to Get PrEP

- **Primary care provider** – Ask if they are comfortable prescribing PrEP.
- **HIV/STI clinics** – Many offer PrEP services with same-day starts.
- **Telehealth services** – Several online providers can prescribe PrEP after a video visit and mail it to you.
- **Pharmacy programs** – In some states, trained pharmacists can prescribe PrEP.

Insurance coverage:

- Most insurance, including Medicaid, covers PrEP at no cost for the medicine itself. Lab tests may have a co-pay depending on your plan.
- **If you're on your parents' insurance:** Your use of PrEP could appear on "Explanation of Benefits" (EOB) forms sent to the policyholder. If privacy is important, talk to your provider or insurance company about confidential communications or consider low-cost clinic programs like Planned Parenthood or local health departments that offer confidential PrEP.

PEP – Post-Exposure Prophylaxis

What it is:

PEP (post-exposure prophylaxis) is an emergency HIV prevention method taken ***after*** you may have been exposed to the virus.

When to use it:

- Condom broke during sex with someone who is known to have or might have HIV
- Had condomless sex with a partner whose status you don't know or know to be positive
- Shared needles or injection equipment with someone at risk or known to be positive
- Needle stick or fluid splash at work (healthcare exposure)

Timing is critical:

- Must start within **72 hours** of exposure (the sooner, the better)
- Taken for **28 days** straight without missing doses

Typical regimen:

- 3 HIV medicines in 2 pills per day
- Most commonly: *Tenofovir disoproxil fumarate with emtricitabine* (Truvada: one pill containing two medicines) + *Raltegravir* or *Dolutegravir* (a second pill containing one medicine)

Possible side effects:

- Nausea, diarrhea, tiredness, or headaches (usually improve after first week)

- Rarely, allergic reactions or liver/kidney problems (your provider will monitor with blood tests)

How to get PEP:

- **Emergency rooms** – fastest option if after hours
- **Urgent care clinics** – many can start PEP same day
- **Some sexual health clinics** – especially in larger cities
- If you need PEP on the weekend or at night, **do not wait**—go to the ER immediately

PEP vs. DoxyPEP – Not the Same Thing

PEP is for HIV prevention after exposure.
DoxyPEP is *doxycycline post-exposure prophylaxis*, an antibiotic taken after condomless sex to help prevent or at least reduce the risk of *bacterial* STIs like syphilis, gonorrhea, and chlamydia—not HIV.

DoxyPEP typical regimen:

- 200 mg of doxycycline (usually 2 pills) taken within 72 hours after sex, ideally within 24 hours
- Possible side effects: nausea, sun sensitivity, stomach upset

Key difference:

- PEP = HIV prevention
- DoxyPEP = bacterial STI prevention

You may be prescribed both if you have a high-risk exposure that puts you at risk for HIV and bacterial STIs.

U=U – Undetectable = Untransmittable

When someone living with HIV takes their medicine every day and their viral load stays so low it can't be measured (undetectable), they **cannot pass HIV sexually**.
This has been proven in thousands of couples with no transmissions over many years.

Real-World Strategy Examples

- **You're HIV-negative and have multiple partners:** Daily oral PrEP or injectable PrEP + regular STI testing; consider DoxyPEP if at high risk for bacterial STIs.
- **You had a one-time high-risk exposure:** Start HIV PEP immediately, consider switching to PrEP after the 28-day course; add DoxyPEP if also exposed to STIs.
- **You have an HIV-positive partner who is undetectable:** No HIV transmission risk from sex, but still test for other STIs regularly.

Key Takeaways

- **PrEP**: Taken before exposure; up to 99% effective against HIV from sex.
- **PEP**: Taken after exposure; start within 72 hours, take for 28 days. **~81% risk reduction** with zidovudine-based PEP after needle-stick injuries. More modern regimens are more potent and better

tolerated, so **true efficacy is likely higher** if started promptly. Most documented PEP failures are linked to **delayed initiation, incomplete adherence**, or **ongoing high-risk exposures during/after PEP**

- **DoxyPEP**: (See Chapter 6) Prevents some bacterial STIs, not HIV. bacterial STIs by **46% (HR 0.54)**. Specifically:
    - **Chlamydia**: reduced by **65%**, though rated low quality evidence
    - **Syphilis**: reduced by **77%**, high quality evidence
    - **Gonorrhea**: no significant reduction (RR 0.90, very low quality evidence) although other studies did show some risk reduction.
- **U=U**: People with undetectable HIV cannot pass it sexually.
- Most insurance covers these; privacy can be an issue on a parent's plan—know your options.

Patient Exercise:

- Do you know where to get PEP at any hour?
- Could you start PrEP this week if you wanted to?
- Do you know of a provider who will prescribe DoxyPEP judgement free?
- If on your parents' insurance, do you know how to request confidential billing?

Chapter 6: Understanding Sexually Transmitted Infections (STIs)

Knowing the Risks, Recognizing the Symptoms, Getting the Right Tests, and Accessing Treatment

Back in Chapter 1, we talked about my friend whose provider was supportive enough to prescribe PrEP and conduct STI testing but didn't know that gonorrhea and chlamydia can infect the throat and rectum as well as the urethra. Since his doctor only tested urine, he had gone for years without ever being screened for anal or oral infections. It was a classic case of both patient and provider wanting to do the right thing but still missing the mark simply because the provider wasn't trained in LGBTQ+ health.

Unfortunately, I've seen provider ignorance play out in even more serious ways. During the COVID epidemic a young resident here in Provincetown developed a lesion on his penis—a classic painless chancre that should have screamed "syphilis" to any clinician familiar with MSM sexual health. He went to our local health center, a place you would expect the staff to be well-versed in these infections. The clinician ordered an RPR blood test, which is a standard syphilis screening test. But here's the catch: in the earliest stages of syphilis, that test often comes back negative. It can take four to six weeks after the appearance of a chancre for the RPR to turn positive. It's simply not a good test for primary syphilis.

The test came back negative, and instead of treating him presumptively—or even explaining the limits of the test—the provider told him it wasn't syphilis and referred him to dermatology. The dermatologist, not suspecting syphilis since the initial provider documented it wasn't a syphilis infection, gave him a steroid cream telling him it was a drug treatment eruption. By the time the real diagnosis came, it wasn't from a clinician—it was through the state's contact tracing after he unknowingly passed syphilis to a partner who was seen by a competent provider. That is when he finally shared the story with me.

This story is frustrating, but it's also the perfect reminder of why *you* need to be informed. Even in practices that should know better, mistakes happen. Knowing what questions to ask, what tests to request, and how window and incubation periods affect results can mean the difference between catching an infection early or missing it altogether.

That's exactly why this chapter exists: to help you understand STIs—not just what they are, but how they're tested, what the limitations of those tests are, and what you should know to advocate for your own care. Because in sexual health, knowledge isn't just power—it's protection.

Many sexually transmitted infections (STIs) can be silent — showing no symptoms for weeks, months, or even years. But even without symptoms, they can cause serious health problems and be passed on to partners. Knowing how STIs work, how they show up in different parts of the body, and how to get accurate testing is essential to protecting your health and your partners.

Window Period vs. Incubation Period

These two terms sound similar but mean very different things:

- **Incubation Period**: The time between when you catch an infection and when symptoms (if any) appear.
  Example: Gonorrhea's incubation period is usually 1–5 days. Syphilis's incubation is about 10–90 days.

- **Window Period**: The time between when you catch an infection and when it can be detected on a test.
  Example: HIV may be detectable on a modern 4th-generation blood test after ~2 weeks, but can take up to 45 days to be certain.

You can have symptoms **before** a test turns positive — or test positive before symptoms appear. That's why timing matters when you get tested after an exposure.

Bacterial STIs

1. Gonorrhea (*Neisseria gonorrhoeae*)

Where it can infect: Penis/urethra, rectum, throat, eyes.

Symptoms vary by site:

- **Urethral**: Usually, burning when urinating, yellow or green discharge, increased urinary frequency but sometimes no symptoms.
- **Rectal**: Usually anal itching, soreness, discharge, bleeding, or feeling like you constantly need to have a bowel movement.

- **Throat**: Usually no symptoms; sometimes sore throat or swollen glands.
- **Eye**: Redness, discharge, swelling (medical emergency).

Incubation period: 1–5 days
Window period for testing: Most NAATs detect within 3–5 days, but testing is most reliable after 7 days.

Testing:

- Ask for **NAAT –(Nucleic Acid Amplification Test) swabs** (e.g. Aptima) from each site you've had contact (genital, rectal, throat). Urine alone is not enough if you've had oral or anal sex.

Treatment:

- CDC recommends **one injection of ceftriaxone 500 mg** (in the buttock or thigh).
- If chlamydia hasn't been ruled out, **doxycycline 100 mg twice daily for 7 days** is also prescribed.
- No sex for 7 days after treatment and until all partners are treated.

□ PATIENT CHECKLIST – Gonorrhea

- ☑ Tell your provider all the sites of sexual contact in the past 60 days (genital, anal, oral).
- ☑ Request **NAAT swabs** from each site — urine alone is not enough if you've had oral or anal sex.
- ☑ Ask when to retest (usually 3 months after treatment).

- ☑ Make sure all partners in the last 60 days are notified and treated.
- ☑ Avoid sex for 7 days after treatment **and** until all partners are treated.

2. Chlamydia (*Chlamydia trachomatis*)

Where it can infect: Penis/urethra, rectum, throat, eyes.
Symptoms vary by site:

- **Urethral**: Burning when urinating, clear or cloudy discharge.
- **Rectal**: Pain, discharge, bleeding, or sometimes nothing at all.
- **Throat**: Usually no symptoms; rarely sore throat.
- **Eye**: Redness, swelling, discharge.

Incubation period: 1–3 weeks
Window period: Most NAAT tests are accurate by day 7 post-exposure.

Testing:

- NAAT swabs from all exposed sites; urine works for urethra but not for rectum or throat.

Treatment:

- **Doxycycline 100 mg twice daily for 7 days**.
- Alternative: Single dose of azithromycin (less effective for rectal infections).
- No sex for 7 days after completion of treatment.

□ **PATIENT CHECKLIST – Chlamydia**

- ☑ Report all possible exposure sites — urethra, rectum, throat.
- ☑ Request **NAAT testing** for each site.
- ☑ Ask if doxycycline is the first-line choice for your infection site.
- ☑ Retest in about 3 months, even if no symptoms.
- ☑ Confirm partners are treated before resuming sex.

3. Syphilis (*Treponema pallidum*)

Stages & symptoms:

- **Primary**: Single painless sore (chancre) at site of infection — genital, anal, oral. Often firm, round, and clean-based. May have swollen lymph nodes nearby. *Important*: Blood tests can be **negative** in early primary syphilis. If you have a typical sore + risk, **treatment should not wait for a positive test**.
- **Secondary**: Rash on palms/soles, mucous patches in mouth, genital wart-like lesions, fever, fatigue.
- **Latent**: No symptoms, but still detectable on tests.
- **Tertiary**: Years later — heart, brain, nerve, or organ damage.

Incubation period: 10–90 days
Window period: RPR/VDRL usually positive 2–6 weeks after infection.

Testing:

- Screening: **RPR** or VDRL.

- Confirmation: **Treponemal test** (e.g., FTA-ABS, TP-PA).
- Ask for both screening and confirmatory testing if risk is high.

Treatment:

- **Primary, secondary, early latent**: One injection of **benzathine penicillin G 2.4 million units.**
- **Late latent or unknown duration**: Weekly injection for 3 weeks.

☐ PATIENT CHECKLIST – Syphilis

- ☑ If you have a sore at a risk site, tell your provider and ask for **treatment immediately** — do not wait for a positive test.
- ☑ Request **RPR/VDRL** and a confirmatory treponemal test.
- ☑ Ask about stage-specific treatment (single vs. three weekly penicillin shots).
- ☑ Schedule follow-up blood tests to ensure your RPR drops after treatment.
- ☑ Avoid sex until treatment is complete and sores are fully healed.

Viral STIs

4. HIV

Symptoms:

- **Acute infection** (2–4 weeks after exposure): Fever, rash, sore throat, swollen lymph nodes, night sweats, diarrhea — often mistaken for flu.
- **Chronic infection**: Can be asymptomatic for years.

Window period:

- 4th-gen tests: Positive as early as 14 days; confirm at 45 days for certainty.

Testing:

- Ask for a **4th-generation HIV antigen/antibody test**.
- If very recent exposure, consider **HIV RNA PCR**.

Treatment:

- Start ART immediately — one pill daily can make viral load undetectable (U=U).

□ PATIENT CHECKLIST – HIV

☑ Request a **4th-generation HIV test** and ask when to repeat it for full accuracy.

- ☑ If recent high-risk exposure (<72 hours), ask if you qualify for **HIV PEP** immediately.

- ☑ If negative but still at risk, discuss starting **HIV PrEP**.
- ☑ If positive, ask to start treatment *the same day.*

5. Herpes (HSV-1 & HSV-2)

Symptoms by site:

- Painful blisters or sores on genitals, anus, or mouth.
- Tingling or itching before outbreaks.
- First outbreak may include fever, body aches, swollen lymph nodes.

Incubation period: 2–12 days
Window period: No standard "window period" — tests depend on whether you have active sores or are using antibody blood tests.

Testing:

- **PCR swab** from an active sore is most accurate.
- Blood tests (type-specific HSV-1/HSV-2 antibodies) can show past exposure, but won't tell you the site or exact timing.

Treatment:

- Antivirals (acyclovir, valacyclovir, famciclovir) shorten outbreaks and reduce frequency.
- Daily suppressive therapy lowers risk of passing herpes to partners.

☐ **PATIENT CHECKLIST – Herpes**

- ☑ If you have sores, request a **PCR swab** from the lesion before it heals.
- ☑ Ask if daily suppressive therapy is right for you.
- ☑ Learn how to recognize early symptoms (tingling, itching) so you can start treatment quickly.
- ☑ Discuss safe-sex strategies to lower the chance of passing herpes to partners.

6. Hepatitis A Virus (HAV)

How it's spread:
Mostly through the fecal–oral route — in sexual contexts, this can include rimming (oral–anal contact) or touching the anal area and then the mouth without washing hands. It can also be spread through contaminated food or water.

Symptoms:

- Fever, fatigue
- Nausea, vomiting, abdominal pain
- Dark urine, pale stools
- Yellowing of eyes or skin (jaundice)
- Some people have no symptoms but can still spread it.

Incubation period: 15–50 days (average ~28)
Window period: HAV IgM antibody appears shortly after symptoms start.

Testing:

- **HAV IgM antibody**: Active/recent infection.
- **HAV IgG antibody**: Past infection or immunity from vaccination.

Treatment:

- Supportive care only — no specific antiviral treatment.
- **Prevention**: Two-dose Hepatitis A vaccine series.

□ **PATIENT CHECKLIST – Hepatitis A**

- ☑ If never vaccinated, request the **Hepatitis A vaccine series**.
- ☑ Ask for HAV IgM/IgG testing if you have jaundice or other symptoms.
- ☑ Practice good hygiene and safe oral–anal contact to avoid reinfection.

7. Hepatitis B Virus (HBV)

How it's spread:
Through blood, semen, vaginal fluids — anal sex is a common route for MSM. Can also be spread by sharing razors, toothbrushes, or needles.

Symptoms:

- Fever, fatigue, loss of appetite
- Nausea, vomiting

- Joint pain
- Dark urine, jaundice
- Many have no symptoms early on.

Incubation period: 45–160 days (average ~90)
Window period: HBV surface antigen appears 1–9 weeks after infection.

Testing:

- **HBsAg** (surface antigen): Active infection.
- **Anti-HBs** (surface antibody): Immunity from past infection or vaccination.
- **Anti-HBc** (core antibody): Past or current infection.

Treatment:

- Acute infection: Supportive care.
- Chronic infection: May need lifelong antiviral therapy.
- **Prevention**: Hepatitis B vaccine series (or 2-dose adult Heplisav-B).

□ PATIENT CHECKLIST – Hepatitis B

- ☑ Ask for the **Hepatitis B vaccine series** if not already immune.
- ☑ Request blood testing (HBsAg, anti-HBs, anti-HBc) to know your status.
- ☑ If positive for chronic HBV, ask about antiviral treatment and liver monitoring.

8. Hepatitis C Virus (HCV)

How it's spread:
Primarily blood-to-blood. Sexual transmission is less common but higher among MSM with HIV and in sexual practices involving bleeding even microscopic amounts of blood which can contaminate toys and other inanimate objects. Sharing items to inject or snort drugs or sharing douching equipment/sex toys can spread HCV.

Symptoms:

- Often none at first.
- Sometimes, Fatigue, nausea, abdominal pain
- Dark urine, rarely jaundice

Incubation period: 2–12 weeks (average 6–7)
Window period:

- HCV RNA PCR: Positive within 1–2 weeks.
- HCV antibody: Positive at 8–11 weeks.

Testing:

- **HCV antibody:** Screening.
- **HCV RNA PCR:** Confirms active infection.

Treatment:

- Direct-acting antivirals cure >95% in 8–12 weeks.
- No vaccine available.

□ PATIENT CHECKLIST – Hepatitis C

- ☑ Request **HCV antibody testing** at least annually if you have ongoing risk.
- ☑ If antibody positive, insist on **HCV RNA testing** to confirm active infection.
- ☑ If positive, ask about direct-acting antivirals (8–12 weeks).
- ☑ Avoid sharing sex toys or engaging in sexual practices that cause bleeding without protection.

Parasitic & Other STIs

9. Trichomoniasis (*Trichomonas vaginalis*)

Symptoms:

- In men: Often none; sometimes urethral irritation, discharge.
- In women: Frothy, foul-smelling discharge, itching.

Incubation period: 5–28 days
Window period: NAAT detects infection as soon as organisms are present.

Testing:

- NAAT is most accurate, wet mount less sensitive.

Treatment:

- **Metronidazole 2 g single dose** or **500 mg twice daily for 7 days**.

- Avoid alcohol during and 24–72 hours after.

PATIENT CHECKLIST – Trichomonas

- ☑ Ask for **NAAT testing** if you have urethral irritation or a partner tests positive.
- ☑ Avoid alcohol if prescribed metronidazole or tinidazole.
- ☑ Retest after treatment if symptoms persist.
- ☑ Make sure partners are treated to avoid reinfection.

Other Sexually Transmitted Intestinal Parasites

Includes *Giardia lamblia*, *Entamoeba histolytica*, *Blastocystis hominis*, and others — spread through oral–anal contact or contaminated food/water. These will be discussed in detail in the next chapter.

PATIENT CHECKLIST – Intestinal Parasites

- ☑ If you have ongoing diarrhea, bloating, or stomach upset, tell your provider about your sexual practices.
- ☑ Ask about stool testing for parasites — if not molecular testing **3 separate specimens** are needed insist on being tested all 3 times.
- ☑ Mention recent travel, group meals, or water exposures.

Prevention Strategies

Doxycycline Post-Exposure Prophylaxis (DoxyPEP)

What it is:
Taking a single antibiotic dose after sex to reduce the chance of certain bacterial STIs.

How it works:
When taken within 72 hours of unprotected sex, doxycycline can prevent chlamydia and syphilis, and reduce gonorrhea risk.

Who it's for:
CDC suggests it for:

- Gay/bisexual men and transgender women
- With an STI in the past year or ongoing high-risk sex

Efficacy:

- Chlamydia: ~65–88% reduction
- Syphilis: ~77–87% reduction
- Gonorrhea: 33–60% reduction, varies by location

How to take it:

- 200 mg (usually two 100 mg tablets)
- As soon as possible after sex, within 72 hours
- No more than once daily

Side effects:

- Nausea, sun sensitivity, stomach upset
- Rare: esophageal irritation (take with water, don't lie down immediately)

Resistance concerns:

- Gonorrhea resistance to tetracyclines exists in some areas; careful monitoring is needed.

Prevention note:

- Does not protect against HIV, herpes, hepatitis.
- Complements, not replaces, condoms, HIV PrEP, and regular STI testing.

✐ PATIENT CHECKLIST – DoxyPEP

- ☑ If you've had an STI in the past year, ask your provider if you qualify for DoxyPEP.
- ☑ Confirm the correct dose: **200 mg within 72 hours after sex** (max once daily).
- ☑ Learn about side effects (nausea, sun sensitivity) and how to reduce them.
- ☑ Continue regular STI testing every 3–6 months while using DoxyPEP.
- ☑ Remember: DoxyPEP does not protect against HIV, herpes, or hepatitis.

Partner Notification: Why It Matters and How to Do It

Telling a partner that you may have exposed them to an STI can feel awkward, scary, or even embarrassing — but it's one of the most important steps in stopping the spread of infection and protecting your own health. Partner notification is not about blame or shame; it's about care, honesty, and public health.

When a partner is informed promptly:

- They can get tested and treated quickly — which reduces the risk of serious complications.
- You lower your chance of being re-infected by them later.
- It helps control STI rates in the community.

Who Needs to Be Told

- **Recent partners** within the look-back period for that STI (your provider can help determine this — for example, 60 days for gonorrhea or chlamydia, up to a year or more for syphilis).
- **Ongoing partners**, even if you haven't had sex recently, if there's a chance of transmission.
- **Casual partners** — if you have a way to contact them.

Ways to Notify

1. **In person or by phone/text**: Direct and personal, best if you have an ongoing relationship.
2. **Through a provider or public health department**: Many clinics and health departments offer confidential partner services where staff contact partners without using your name.
3. **Using an anonymous notification service**:
   - Websites like tellyourpartner.org or dontspreadit.com send anonymous texts or emails.

4. **Dating app notifications**: Some apps have built-in STI notification features.

What to Say

Keep it short, factual, and free of blame. For example:

"I recently tested positive for [STI name]. You should get tested and treated. It can be easily cured/managed if caught early. Here's a clinic number or link for info."

If You're Worried About Safety

If you fear your partner might react with violence or harassment, use an anonymous notification option or have your provider or health department make the contact.

🔊 PATIENT CHECKLIST – Partner Notification

- ☑ Ask your provider which partners need to be told and the time frame for your infection.
- ☑ Choose the safest method for you (direct, provider-assisted, anonymous).
- ☑ Share clear, factual information about the STI, and where to get tested/treated.
- ☑ If you're worried about your safety, let your provider or health department handle notification.
- ☑ Avoid sexual contact with any untreated partner until they complete treatment and are cleared.

Summary Table: Common Sexually Transmitted Infections at a Glance

Infection	Main Sites	Incubation	Window Period	Testing	Treatment / Prevention
Gonorrhea	Genital, rectal, throat, eye	1–5 d	3–7 d	NAAT site-specific	Ceftriaxone injection
Chlamydia	Genital, rectal, throat, eye	1–21 d	7 d	NAAT site-specific	Doxycycline 7 days
Syphilis	Genital, anal, oral, systemic	10–90 d	2–6 w	RPR + treponemal test	Penicillin injection
HIV	Blood, systemic	2–4 w (acute)	2–6 w	4th-gen ± RNA PCR	Lifelong ART
Herpes	Genital, anal, oral	2–12 d	N/A	PCR from sore	Antivirals
Trichomonas	Genital	5–28 d	7 d	NAAT	Metronidazole
Hepatitis A	Liver/systemic	15–50 d	2-6 weeks	HAV IgM and IgG	Supportive care; vaccine

Infection	Main Sites	Incubation	Window Period	Testing	Treatment / Prevention
Hepatitis B	Liver/systemic	45–160 d	1–9 weeks	HBsAg, anti-HBs, anti-HBc	Antivirals for chronic; vaccine
Hepatitis C	Liver/systemic	2–12 w	1–11 weeks	HCV Ab + RNA PCR	8–12 wk antivirals; no vaccine

Chapter 7:

Sexually Transmitted Gastroenteropathies

(Stomach Infections)

Intestinal Infections, Proctitis, and Other Gut Conditions from Sexual Transmission

Over six years ago, I wrote a blog post for gay men that hit a nerve. It originated out of my practice experience in finding that a surprising number of men who had either been told by a provider or diagnosed themselves with *lactose intolerance*, *food allergies*, or *irritable bowel syndrome (IBS)* weren't dealing with digestive problems at all—they were living with sexually transmitted bacterial or protozoal infections of the gut. Many of these men had spent years putting up with diarrhea, bloating, frequent foul-smelling gas, and other digestive symptoms while seeing provider after provider who never considered that sex—not dairy—was the cause.

Here's the problem: not every parasite is considered "disease-causing" in the general population, but in men who have sex with men, certain organisms that might otherwise be written off as "harmless" can wreak havoc. Additionally, even parasites that are disease causing are much less often seen in non-MSM patients because they have different risk profiles. Beyond parasites, **I've seen many men with *lymphogranuloma venereum (LGV) proctitis* misdiagnosed with Crohn's disease**—a serious mistake that delayed treatment and caused needless suffering.

These stories matter because they show why *you* need at least a basic understanding of sexually transmitted gastroenteropathies a.k.a stomach problems. Even if your provider doesn't bring it up—or doesn't know to look for it—you'll be able to ask the right questions and advocate for yourself. Knowledge can save years of frustration, misdiagnosis, and the very real health risks that come from untreated infections.

Why This Chapter Matters

When people think about sexually transmitted infections, they often think about genitals — not the gut. But many infections can be spread through sexual practices, especially oral–anal contact (also called "rimming"), anal sex, or sharing sex toys. These can cause chronic diarrhea, bloating, abdominal pain, rectal bleeding, or systemic illness.

Some gut infections are **bacterial or parasitic**, others are **viral**, and some involve **inflammatory damage** that can mimic unrelated diseases like Crohn's. As I described in the opening of this chapter because many healthcare providers receive minimal training in sexually transmitted gastroenteropathies, symptoms can be misdiagnosed or dismissed, leaving patients to suffer for months or even years.

1. Lymphogranuloma Venereum (LGV) Proctitis

Cause: Certain aggressive strains (serovars L1, L2, L3) of *Chlamydia trachomatis.*

Symptoms:

- Rectal pain and bleeding
- Mucus discharge from the rectum
- Tenesmus (feeling you constantly need to have a bowel movement)
- Sometimes fever, malaise, or painful swollen lymph nodes in the groin

- Chronic untreated LGV can cause scarring and strictures of the rectum

Why it's often missed:
LGV proctitis can look almost identical to **Crohn's disease** — both on symptoms and even on colonoscopy biopsy. In fact:

- Some patients have been mistakenly diagnosed with Crohn's and started on **immunosuppressive therapy**, which can worsen LGV.
- Standard STI testing for *Chlamydia* doesn't always check for LGV serotypes unless specifically requested.
- Pathology reports from biopsies may not mention chlamydia unless special stains are done.

If you've been diagnosed with Crohn's disease but are a sexually active man who has receptive anal sex, ask:

- Were LGV serotype antibody tests done?
- Was *Chlamydia trachomatis* tested from rectal swabs by NAAT?
- Were colonoscopy biopsy samples stained specifically for chlamydia or **Mycoplasma genitalium** (which can also cause proctitis)?

Treatment:

- **Doxycycline 100 mg twice daily for 21 days** (longer than regular chlamydia treatment).

□ **PATIENT CHECKLIST – LGV Proctitis**

- ☑ If you have rectal pain, bleeding, or Crohn's-like symptoms, ask for rectal NAAT for chlamydia and LGV serovar testing.
- ☑ If diagnosed with Crohn's, confirm whether biopsies were stained for chlamydia and mycoplasma.
- ☑ Ask if LGV antibody testing is available.
- ☑ Avoid anal sex until treatment is complete and follow-up testing is negative.

2. Intestinal Protozoa and Parasites

Many providers were taught that some intestinal organisms found on stool testing — like *Blastocystis hominis* and *Endolimax nana* — are harmless "commensals." While that's true for many people, in **symptomatic patients** (especially MSM) these can be **pathogenic** and cause:

- Chronic diarrhea
- Abdominal cramping
- Bloating and gas
- Fatigue and weight loss

Blastocystis hominis:

- Can cause intermittent or persistent diarrhea.
- Symptoms sometimes improve with treatment (metronidazole, nitazoxanide).

Endolimax nana:

- Often dismissed, but in some people linked to GI symptoms.
- Treatment may include metronidazole.

Why patients are told "it's not causing your problems": Some labs don't differentiate between colonization and disease, and providers may be using outdated teaching. In high-risk sexual exposures, these organisms *should* be considered possible causes.

☐ **PATIENT CHECKLIST – Blastocystis & Endolimax**

- ☑ If diagnosed with these parasites and you have symptoms, ask about treatment options — don't accept "it's harmless" without discussion.
- ☑ Request stool PCR or ova/parasite testing for multiple days (3 samples often increases detection).
- ☑ Tell your provider about your sexual history so they understand risk of pathogenic infection.

3. Brachyspira (Intestinal Spirochetosis)

Cause: *Brachyspira aalborgi* or *Brachyspira pilosicoli* — spiral-shaped bacteria that infect the colon lining.

Symptoms:

- Chronic diarrhea
- Mucus in stool
- Abdominal discomfort
- Sometimes no symptoms at all

Why it's hard to diagnose:

- Rarely detected by standard stool PCR panels.

- Often found only on colon biopsy under special stains.

Treatment:

- Metronidazole is most often used, though data is limited.

□ **PATIENT CHECKLIST – Brachyspira**

- ☑ If you have chronic unexplained diarrhea and normal stool tests, ask if colonoscopy with special staining for Brachyspira is appropriate.
- ☑ Discuss empiric treatment options if biopsy confirms infection.

4. Other Sexually Transmitted Gut Pathogens

These include:

- **Giardia lamblia** — common cause of diarrhea from oral–anal contact; often treated with metronidazole or tinidazole.
- **Entamoeba histolytica** — can cause severe colitis or liver abscesses; requires specific anti-amoebic therapy.
- **Campylobacter, Shigella, Salmonella** — bacterial gut infections that can be sexually transmitted; treated with antibiotics in some cases.

Note: Many of these require **multiple stool specimens** to detect, as shedding can be intermittent.

□ PATIENT CHECKLIST – General GI STI Testing

- ☑ If symptomatic, request stool testing for ova/parasites, bacterial cultures, and PCR for protozoa and bacteria.
- ☑ Give multiple stool specimens on different days to improve detection.
- ☑ Mention sexual practices that might increase GI infection risk.

5. Long-Term Complication: Exocrine Pancreatic Insufficiency (EPI)

Some people who have prolonged, untreated intestinal infections go on to develop **EPI** — where the pancreas doesn't make enough digestive enzymes. This leads to:

- Chronic diarrhea with greasy, floating, foul-smelling stools
- Weight loss
- Nutrient deficiencies

The good news: In many cases caused by infection, EPI gradually resolves over 6–12 months after the infection is treated — but in the meantime, enzyme replacement therapy can be life-changing.

Testing:

- **Fecal elastase test** — measures pancreatic enzyme output.

Also important for HIV-positive patients:

- EPI is more common in people with HIV on ART, and it's often missed.

□ PATIENT CHECKLIST – Exocrine Pancreatic Insufficiency

- ☑ If you've had long-term gut infections and now have greasy stools, weight loss, or ongoing diarrhea, ask for a **fecal elastase test**.
- ☑ If EPI is diagnosed, ask about prescription pancreatic enzyme replacement until function recovers.
- ☑ If you have HIV, discuss EPI screening with your provider even without a known gut infection history.

⚠□ PATIENT CHECKLIST – Misdiagnosis Alert

- ☑ Don't accept an IBS, lactose intolerance, or food allergy diagnosis without ruling out infection.
- ☑ Ask for **PCR-based stool testing** covering bacteria, parasites, and viruses.
- ☑ Provide **three separate stool specimens** collected on different days for ova/parasite exams.
- ☑ Confirm whether colonoscopy biopsies were stained for ***Brachyspira* (intestinal spirochetosis)**.
- ☑ If your provider says certain parasites like *Blastocystis* or *Endolimax* are harmless, ask if treatment is still reasonable given your symptoms if they say no insist or find another provider.

A Note on Exocrine Pancreatic Insufficiency (EPI)

Sometimes, after a parasite or other intestinal infection has been treated and eradicated, symptoms don't immediately go away. Many men continue to experience diarrhea, bloating, and gas for weeks or months. One reason is that chronic gut inflammation can disrupt the pancreas, leading to **exocrine pancreatic insufficiency (EPI)**.

When this happens, your pancreas isn't producing enough digestive enzymes to break down fats, proteins, and carbs properly. The result? Food moves through your system only partially digested—leaving you with lingering symptoms that feel a lot like the original infection.

If you've had a gut parasite or bacterial infection and still don't feel right after treatment, ask your provider to order a **fecal elastase test**. This simple stool test can show whether your pancreas is underperforming. If EPI is present, you may need to take **digestive enzyme supplements** for a while.

The good news is that in many cases the pancreas recovers once inflammation settles down, and your enzyme production goes back to normal. But even if it doesn't, enzyme replacement therapy works very well. With treatment, you'll be back to enjoying your whey protein, ice cream, and cheese without all the drama.

Closing Thoughts

Sexually transmitted gastroenteropathies can be complex, often overlapping in symptoms and requiring specialized tests to diagnose. Many are missed or dismissed because providers rely on outdated teaching or do not take detailed sexual histories.

Far too often, men who have sex with men are told — or tell themselves — that their chronic diarrhea, bloating, or abdominal pain is due to irritable bowel syndrome (IBS), lactose intolerance, or a vague "food allergy." While those conditions are real, in many cases the actual cause is an undiagnosed infectious gastroenteropathy.

Unless you have been:

- Tested with **PCR-based stool testing**,
- Provided **three separate stool specimens on different days** for ova and parasite examination, **and**
- Specifically been evaluated for *Brachyspira* (intestinal spirochetosis) on colon biopsy,

you cannot confidently rule out an infectious cause. Jumping to an IBS or food intolerance label without this work-up risks delaying effective treatment — sometimes for years. If treating these doesn't solve the problem check fecal elastase more often than not- that's the remaining issue.

As a patient, your voice matters — asking for specific tests, clarifying how samples are processed, and insisting on follow-up can make the difference between months of suffering and quick recovery.

Chapter 8

HPV, Anal Pap & Cancer Prevention

Understanding the Human Papillomavirus and Protecting Your Health

If you were a gay man coming of age in the '70s or '80s, chances are you had a poster of Farrah Fawcett somewhere—or at least you knew someone who did. She was the very definition of a gay icon: dazzling smile, feathered hair, and that blend of beauty and charisma that made her unforgettable. But Farrah's story took a devastating turn when she was diagnosed with **anal cancer**, an often HPV-associated cancer that ultimately took her life at just 62.

Here's why that matters for us. Anal cancer, like cervical cancer, is often driven by persistent infection with **human papillomavirus (HPV)**. Women have long benefitted from cervical Pap smears, which catch precancerous changes early, before they become life-threatening. Gay and bisexual men, however, face **similar risks of anal cancer**, yet screening and prevention efforts have lagged far behind. In fact, we still don't do a great job of screening women for HPV-associated anal cancers—and for MSM, the system has often done little to nothing.

That's the serious part. The "fun" part—if you can call it that—is that prevention really does work. Anal Pap smears and high-resolution anoscopy may not sound glamorous (Farrah probably wouldn't have put *that* on a poster), but they save lives. Add to that the HPV vaccine—which many adults still don't realize is an option—and suddenly we have real tools to stop a preventable cancer in its tracks.

Farrah's story is a reminder that cancer doesn't care about fame, beauty, or sexual orientation. But our community can learn from her loss. For MSM, being proactive about HPV vaccination, talking to your provider about anal Pap screening, and pushing for prevention isn't just medical housekeeping. It's how we protect our health, our futures, and yes—our ability to keep enjoying life, hair feathered or not.

Why This Chapter Matters

Human papillomavirus (HPV) is the most common sexually transmitted infection in the world. Almost everyone who is sexually active will be exposed at some point — but for most people, the body clears the virus naturally. In some cases, however, certain strains of HPV can lead to genital warts or, more seriously, cancer.

For gay, bisexual, and other men who have sex with men (MSM), the risk of anal cancer is significantly higher — especially for men living with HIV. This makes prevention, early detection, and treatment essential parts of your sexual health plan.

HPV Basics

- **What it is**: A group of over 100 viruses. Some cause warts; others cause cancers.
- **High-risk types**: HPV-16 and HPV-18 are linked to most anal, cervical, and some head-and-neck cancers.
- **Low-risk types**: HPV-6 and HPV-11 cause most genital warts.

How it spreads:

- Skin-to-skin sexual contact — not just penetration.
- Oral, anal, and genital contact.
- Can be passed even when no warts or symptoms are visible.

HPV in Men Who Have Sex With Men

- Anal HPV infection is common — studies show **over 60%** of HIV-negative MSM and **over 90%** of HIV-positive MSM have anal HPV at some point.
- Anal cancer rates among MSM are **20–40 times higher** than in the general male population.
- Among HIV-positive MSM, anal cancer incidence can exceed **80 cases per 100,000 men per year** — comparable to cervical cancer rates before Pap testing was routine in women.

Symptoms of HPV Infection

Most HPV infections cause **no symptoms** and clear on their own.
Possible symptoms:

- Small bumps or growths (warts) on the penis, anus, scrotum, groin, or in the throat.
- Changes in skin texture or color in genital/anal areas.
- Anal bleeding, pain, or itching (can be caused by warts or precancer).

HPV Vaccination

Gardasil 9 protects against:

- High-risk types: 16, 18, 31, 33, 45, 52, 58
- Low-risk types: 6 and 11

Who should get vaccinated:

- Recommended for all people through age 26.
- Ages 27–45: Can still benefit; discuss with your provider.
- Works best before HPV exposure, but can still protect against types you haven't yet acquired.

Schedule:

- Under 15: 2 doses (0 and 6–12 months).
- Age 15 or older: 3 doses (0, 1–2 months, 6 months).

✔ PATIENT CHECKLIST – HPV Vaccination

- ☑ Ask your provider if you've received **all recommended doses** of Gardasil 9.
- ☑ If unvaccinated and under 45, discuss starting the series.
- ☑ Keep your vaccination record for future reference.

Anal Cancer Risk and Screening

Risk factors:

- HIV infection
- History of anal warts
- Persistent infection with high-risk HPV
- Smoking

Anal Pap test:

- Similar to a cervical Pap smear but done on anal tissue.
- Detects abnormal cells caused by HPV.
- Recommended annually for HIV-positive MSM and every 2–3 years for sexually active HIV-negative MSM.

High-resolution anoscopy (HRA):

- If the anal Pap shows abnormal cells, HRA is a follow up test that uses a magnifying scope to closely examine and biopsy suspicious areas.
- During the procedure they can also treat precancerous lesions before they progress preventing cancer from ever occurring.

□ PATIENT CHECKLIST – Anal Cancer Screening

- ☑ Ask for **anal Pap testing** based on your risk profile.
- ☑ If you have HIV, request annual screening.
- ☑ If your anal Pap is abnormal, ask about referral for **high-resolution anoscopy**.

- ☑ Report any anal bleeding, pain, or lumps promptly.

Vetting a Provider for Anal Pap and HRA

Not every provider who offers an anal Pap does it well — and not every abnormal result gets managed correctly. Here's what to know:

Signs your provider knows what they're doing:

- They use a moistened swab inserted into the anal canal, rotating to collect cells from all sides.
- They do both cytology and HPV testing on the swab.
- They explain how often you should repeat the test based on your results and risk factors.
- If your Pap is abnormal, they refer you to a provider who does **high-resolution anoscopy (HRA)**, not just a colonoscopy.

Why colonoscopy isn't enough:

- Colonoscopy looks for polyps and tumors in the colon — it's not designed to detect HPV-related precancer in the anal canal.
- Many anal cancers start at the squamocolumnar junction (just inside the anus) — this area is best examined with HRA.

Questions to ask before scheduling HRA:

1. **How many HRAs do you perform each month?** More procedures = more skill.
2. **Where did you train to do HRA?** Look for training through reputable programs such as the International Anal Neoplasia Society (IANS) or large teaching hospitals with anal dysplasia programs.
3. **Do you use anesthesia?** HRA is typically done in an exam room **without** sedation — if a provider insists on general anesthesia for routine HRA, that's a red flag.
4. **Do you perform biopsies and treatment during the same visit?** This is important so you don't have to schedule a second procedure.
5. **Do you follow International Anal Neoplasia Society guidelines?** This helps ensure your care is evidence-based.

🔍 PATIENT CHECKLIST – Vetting Anal Pap & HRA Providers

- ☑ Ask how your anal Pap will be collected and how often it's repeated.
- ☑ If abnormal, confirm referral for **high-resolution anoscopy** (not colonoscopy).
- ☑ Ask how many HRAs the provider does monthly.
- ☑ Ask **where they trained** to do HRA and whether they follow International Anal Neoplasia Society guidelines.
- ☑ Ask if they do biopsies and treatment in the same session.

- ☑ Ask if they use anesthesia — be cautious if they recommend general anesthesia for routine HRA.

Oral HPV and Throat Cancer

HPV can also infect the throat and cause cancers at the base of the tongue or tonsils. These cancers are increasing in men. **Prevention tips**:

- HPV vaccination
- Regular dental/oral check-ups
- Reporting persistent sore throat, lumps, or voice changes

Myths & Facts About HPV

Myth: HPV only affects women.
Fact: HPV can cause cancers in men too — especially anal, penile, and throat cancers.

Myth: The HPV vaccine isn't useful if you're already sexually active.
Fact: Even if you've been exposed to some types, the vaccine protects against others.

Myth: Condoms prevent all HPV transmission.
Fact: Condoms lower the risk but don't fully protect against HPV since it spreads by skin-to-skin contact.

Myth: Anal Pap tests are only needed if you have symptoms.
Fact: Most precancerous changes have no symptoms — screening finds them early.

□ PATIENT CHECKLIST – HPV Prevention

- ☑ Complete HPV vaccination series.
- ☑ Use condoms and barriers for oral–anal sex if you are worried about HPV spread.
- ☑ Keep up with anal Pap testing and follow-up exams.
- ☑ Avoid smoking to lower cancer risk it has synergy with HPV to increase risk.

Closing Thoughts

HPV is extremely common, but serious complications can be prevented. For MSM — particularly those living with HIV — proactive prevention and screening are essential. With vaccination, regular anal Pap testing, and prompt treatment of precancer, the vast majority of HPV-related cancers can be avoided.

Chapter 9: Hepatitis A, B & C

Protecting Your Liver and Your Health

When most people think about PrEP, they think about HIV prevention. But here's something you may not know: some PrEP medicines also affect hepatitis B, albeit they <u>DO NOT</u> prevent HBV infection while others don't touch HBV infection at all. That difference can be a very big deal.

Right now, there are two oral forms of PrEP and two injectable forms available. The oral versions (which contain tenofovir) do double duty—preventing HIV and also keeping hepatitis B under control if you have it. The injectable versions prevent HIV just as effectively, but they do not treat hepatitis B. That means if someone has hepatitis B and doesn't know it, oral PrEP is quietly holding the virus in check. If they suddenly stop oral PrEP—say, to switch to an injectable—hepatitis B can "wake up" and flare. A flare is when the virus rebounds strongly, causing major liver inflammation and, in some cases, life-threatening liver damage.

This is not just a theory. A patient in New York City recently experienced a severe hepatitis B flare after stopping oral PrEP, and it was so aggressive that he required a liver transplant. Situations like this underline why it is essential that your provider knows how to test for hepatitis B before you start PrEP or change PrEP regimens.

Hepatitis C is a little different. Neither oral nor injectable PrEP has any effect on it. If you have hepatitis C, you won't get a flare when you change PrEP types—but you also won't get any protection from the medication. Untreated, hepatitis C can silently cause liver scarring and cirrhosis over time. The good news is that hepatitis C is now curable with a short course of oral medications—usually 8 to 12 weeks.

Both hepatitis B and hepatitis C can be transmitted sexually, and hepatitis C in particular spreads easily when men share drug-using equipment like needles, syringes, cookers, or rinse water. That's why testing for these infections is just as important as testing for HIV when you start PrEP.

Knowing your hepatitis B and C status—and making sure your provider tests you correctly—protects you not just from HIV, but from serious, and sometimes life-threatening, liver complications. This is knowledge that can literally save your liver.

Why This Chapter Matters

Your liver is one of the most important organs in your body — it processes nutrients, filters toxins, and supports your immune system. Hepatitis viruses cause inflammation of the liver, which can range from mild illness to life-threatening disease.

For gay, bisexual, and other men who have sex with men (MSM), the risk of hepatitis A, B, and C is higher due to certain sexual practices, shared drug equipment, and other exposure routes. The good news: hepatitis A and B can largely be **prevented with vaccines**, and hepatitis C can now be **cured** in most people.

Hepatitis A (HAV)

How it spreads:
HAV spreads through the **fecal–oral route** — meaning microscopic amounts of stool (poop) get into the mouth. In sexual contexts, this often happens with oral–anal contact ("rimming") or touching the anal area and then the mouth without washing hands. It can also spread via contaminated food or water.

Symptoms:

- Fever, fatigue
- Nausea, vomiting, abdominal pain
- Loss of appetite
- Dark urine, pale stools
- Yellowing of eyes or skin (jaundice)

Some people — especially children — may have no symptoms but can still spread the virus.

Incubation period: 15–50 days (average ~28)
Window period for testing: HAV IgM antibody becomes positive soon after symptoms start.

Testing:

- **HAV IgM antibody**: Shows current or recent infection.
- **HAV IgG antibody**: Shows immunity from past infection or vaccination.

Treatment:

- No specific antiviral — illness usually resolves on its own.

- Supportive care (rest, fluids, avoiding alcohol and liver-toxic drugs).

Prevention:

- Two-dose Hepatitis A vaccine series (safe, effective, and provides long-lasting immunity).
- If you're unsure whether you're immune, **ask for a hepatitis A IgG titer** to check.
- Keep a record of your immune status in your medical chart.

💉 PATIENT CHECKLIST – Hepatitis

- ☑ If never vaccinated, request the Hepatitis A vaccine series.
- ☑ If unsure of your immune status, request a **HAV IgG titer** and record results in your medical records.
- ☑ Ask for HAV IgM/IgG testing if you have jaundice, dark urine, or flu-like illness with stomach upset.
- ☑ Practice good hygiene and safe oral–anal contact to reduce risk.

Hepatitis B (HBV)

How it spreads:
HBV spreads through **blood, semen, vaginal fluids, and other body fluids**. Sexual contact is a major route for MSM. It can also be passed by sharing razors, toothbrushes, or needles.

Symptoms (acute infection):

- Fever, fatigue
- Loss of appetite
- Nausea, vomiting
- Joint pain
- Dark urine, jaundice
- Many have no symptoms at all

Risks of chronic infection:

- Cirrhosis (scarring of the liver)
- Liver cancer

Incubation period: 45–160 days (average ~90)
Window period: HBV surface antigen appears 1–9 weeks after infection.

Testing:

- **HBsAg** (surface antigen): Active infection.
- **Anti-HBs** (surface antibody): Immunity from past infection or vaccination.
- **Anti-HBc** (core antibody): Past or current infection.

Treatment:

- Acute infection: Usually resolves on its own; supportive care.
- Chronic infection: May require lifelong antiviral medication to prevent liver damage.

Prevention:

- Hepatitis B vaccine series (three doses, or two doses with Heplisav-B for adults).

- Combination Hepatitis A/B vaccine is also available.
- If you're unsure whether you're immune, request a **Hepatitis B surface antibody (anti-HBs) titer**.
- If you are immune, record the titer result in your medical records.
- For people at ongoing risk, consider **rechecking anti-HBs titers every few years** — a booster may be needed if immunity wanes.
- **If you have completed the standard Hepatitis B vaccine series but your titer shows you are still not immune**, ask your provider about **Dynavax Heplisav-B**.
    - **Why?** Heplisav-B is a newer, two-dose vaccine for adults that uses a different adjuvant (immune booster) than the older vaccines. Studies show it produces a stronger immune response — especially in people who did not respond to traditional Hepatitis B vaccination.

💉 PATIENT CHECKLIST – Hepatitis B

- ☑ Ask for the Hepatitis B vaccine if not immune.
- ☑ Request blood testing (HBsAg, anti-HBs, anti-HBc) to know your status.
- ☑ If unsure of your immune status, request a **Hepatitis B surface antibody titer** and record results in your medical records.
- ☑ If at continued risk, **recheck anti-HBs titers every few years**.
- ☑ If vaccinated but **not immune**, ask about **Dynavax Heplisav-B** for a stronger response.

- ☑ If chronic HBV is found, ask about antiviral treatment and regular liver monitoring.

Hepatitis C (HCV)

How it spreads:
Primarily **blood-to-blood contact**. While sexual transmission risk is lower for most people, it's higher in MSM who are HIV-positive, have other STIs, or engage in sexual practices that cause bleeding (fisting, rough anal sex, sharing sex toys). Sharing needles or drug equipment — including for recreational drugs — is also a major risk.

Symptoms:

- Often none in early infection
- Fatigue, nausea, abdominal pain
- Dark urine, jaundice (less common early)

Risks of chronic infection:

- Cirrhosis
- Liver cancer

Incubation period: 2–12 weeks (average 6–7)
Window period:

- HCV RNA PCR: Detectable in 1–2 weeks
- HCV antibody: Detectable at 8–11 weeks

Testing:

- **HCV antibody test:** Screens for past or current infection.
- **HCV RNA PCR:** Confirms if the virus is active.

Treatment:

- Direct-acting antivirals cure >95% of cases, often in just 8–12 weeks.

Prevention:

- No vaccine available.
- Reduce risk by avoiding shared needles/equipment, using condoms and gloves for high-risk sexual activities, and cleaning sex toys between partners.

☐ PATIENT CHECKLIST – Hepatitis C

- ☑ Ask for HCV antibody testing at least annually if you have ongoing risk.
- ☑ If antibody-positive, insist on HCV RNA testing to confirm active infection.
- ☑ If positive, discuss antiviral treatment options — cure rates are very high.
- ☑ Avoid sharing sex toys or engaging in practices that cause bleeding without protection.

Myths & Facts About Hepatitis A, B & C

Myth: You can't get hepatitis A, B, or C from sex.
Fact: All three can be sexually transmitted. Hepatitis A and B are more easily spread through sexual contact, while hepatitis C risk is higher with certain practices (rough anal sex, fisting, sharing sex toys, other STIs).

Myth: If you feel fine, you can't have hepatitis.
Fact: Many people have no symptoms for years while the virus silently damages their liver.

Myth: If you've been vaccinated for hepatitis B, you're automatically immune.
Fact: Some people don't respond to the vaccine. You need a **titer test** to confirm immunity. If you're not immune, Heplisav-B can often work when the older vaccines did not.

Myth: Hepatitis C can't be cured.
Fact: Modern treatments cure over 95% of people in just 8–12 weeks.

Myth: You only need to be tested for hepatitis once.
Fact: If you have ongoing risk, you may need **periodic testing** — especially for hepatitis C.

□ PATIENT CHECKLIST – Hepatitis Prevention & Testing

- ☑ Complete Hepatitis A and B vaccinations — confirm immunity with titer testing.
- ☑ If Hep B vaccination failed, ask about Dynavax's Heplisav-B.
- ☑ Test for hepatitis C at least once; repeat if at ongoing risk.
- ☑ Avoid sharing needles, personal hygiene items, or sex toys without cleaning.
- ☑ Use condoms and barriers for oral–if not immune to hepatitis A and B and there's risk.
- ☑ Record your immune status in your medical records and recheck periodically if you're at risk.

Chapter 10:

Sex Practices & Fetishes 101 – Consent, Hygiene, and Respect

Over my 22 years of practice, I've learned that what patients don't share with their providers can sometimes be as important as what they do. Three patients I know of have died from fisting and one of them was a patient I actually saw while I was a student. The other two were patients of my mentor. One ruptured an undiagnosed aortic aneurysm during play. The other two suffered colon perforations and died of sepsis before they could reach the emergency room.

None of these men had shared that they were into fisting and back in those days it was a rare behavior. The partner of one of the men was almost charged by the NY district attorney's office with manslaughter. I don't know if disclosure to their primary care doctor or in the case of my patient, to me, would have changed any outcomes—but I do know this: when I share these stories with current patients who are into fisting, they are almost always shocked. Many don't realize that something they thought of as adventurous, and erotic could turn deadly.

That's why this chapter exists. Not to shame or sensationalize, but to provide clear, accurate information. Because whether we're talking about fisting, role play, BDSM, or any other fetish, **knowledge is power**. The more you understand about your own body, about risks and safe practices, and about how to communicate openly and respectfully with partners, the safer and more fulfilling your experiences can be.

So let's talk honestly—about consent, about hygiene, about safety, and about respect. Because pleasure should never cost a life.

Why This Chapter Matters

Sexual expression comes in many forms. Whether you enjoy traditional sex, kink, fetish play, group encounters, or BDSM, understanding how to navigate these activities with **consent, hygiene, and respect** can make them safer, more pleasurable, and less likely to cause harm.

This chapter is **not** here to shame or limit you — it's here to empower you with knowledge so you can make informed choices that protect your health, your partners, and your enjoyment.

Consent: The Non-Negotiable Foundation

Consent is the enthusiastic, informed, and ongoing agreement to participate in sexual activity. Without it, sex is assault. With it, sex can be mutually satisfying and respectful.

Key principles of consent:

- **Freely given** – no coercion, manipulation, or pressure.
- **Informed** – everyone knows what's on the table (and what's not).
- **Enthusiastic** – participants genuinely want to do it.
- **Specific** – agreeing to one act doesn't mean agreeing to others.
- **Ongoing** – can be withdrawn at any time.

Special considerations for kink & fetish play:

- Negotiate activities before starting.
- Use **safe words** — a pre-agreed word or signal that means “stop” immediately.
- Check in during scenes — especially if power exchange or restraints are involved.

□ PATIENT CHECKLIST – Practicing Consent

- ☑ Discuss boundaries and interests before play.
- ☑ Agree on safe words or signals.
- ☑ Respect “no” without question or persuasion.
- ☑ Recheck consent during play, especially in intense or emotional scenes.
- ☑ Debrief afterward — check in emotionally and physically.

Hygiene: Keeping It Clean Without Killing the Mood

Cleanliness matters for both health and pleasure, but “clean” doesn’t mean “sterile.” Over-washing or using harsh products can cause irritation and increase infection risk.

General hygiene tips:

- Shower before play if possible — or use wipes if you can’t.

- Trim nails and remove sharp jewelry if they may be involved in contact.
- Clean toys before and after use with soap and water or toy-safe cleaner.
- Use condoms or barriers for easier cleanup and reduced STI risk.

Anal play hygiene:

- Anal sex does not require being "enema clean" for safety — but some people prefer it for comfort or aesthetics.
- If using enemas, use warm (not hot) water and avoid repeated deep douching before sex — this can irritate tissue and increase STI susceptibility.
- Avoid soaps or harsh chemicals internally.

□ **PATIENT CHECKLIST – Hygiene & Safety**

- ☑ Wash hands and genitals before and after play.
- ☑ Clean toys between partners or use condoms on them.
- ☑ Avoid sharing douching equipment.
- ☑ Check lube compatibility with condoms and toys (oil can degrade latex).
- ☑ Dry gear fully before storage to avoid mold or bacteria growth.

Respect: The Culture of Good Play

Respect in sexual encounters means honoring your partner's boundaries, body, and dignity.

Key points:

- Don't assume someone's interests based on appearance or orientation.
- Never "out" someone's sexual practices to others without permission.
- Understand that kinks and fetishes are often deeply personal — treat disclosure as private and privileged.
- Be aware of power imbalances — age, experience, physical strength, or relationship dynamics can all affect how comfortable someone feels saying "no."

Common Sex Practices & Fetishes — Health Considerations

Practice/Fetish	What It Involves	Health Considerations
Anal sex	Penetration of the anus with penis, fingers, toys	Use plenty of lube, start slow, use condoms to prevent STIs, be mindful of tissue fragility
Rimming	Oral contact with the anus	Barrier use (dental dam), hygiene, hepatitis A vaccination
Fisting	Hand or fist insertion into anus or vagina	Use lots of lube, trim nails, go slow, use gloves

Practice/Fetish	What It Involves	Health Considerations
		to reduce STI risk
Watersports	Urine play	Low infection risk if healthy, higher with STIs/UTI; avoid large amounts of concentrated urine
BDSM	Bondage, discipline, dominance/submission, sadomasochism	Negotiate clearly, avoid nerve and blood vessel compression, aftercare matters
Electroplay	Sexual use of electrical stimulation devices	Use only equipment made for erotic use; avoid if you have heart conditions or pacemakers
Group sex / sex parties	Multiple partners in one encounter	Plan for safer sex supplies, STI testing afterward, respect boundaries

Fisting & Large Toy Play — Pleasure with Caution

Fisting and the use of oversized toys can be intensely pleasurable for some people, but these activities carry higher physical risks than most sexual practices and have resulted in deaths. Awareness and preparation are key to keeping them safe.

What It Involves

- **Fisting**: Insertion of an entire hand (and sometimes forearm) into the rectum or vagina.
- **Large toy play**: Insertion of toys that are significantly wider than average penis girth.

Both require **extensive preparation**, patience, and constant communication.

Risks — Common & Rare

- **Minor tearing** of the anal or vaginal tissue (common without enough lube or warm-up).
- **Hemorrhoids or fissures** from stretching.
- **STI transmission** (especially if gloves or condoms aren't used).
- **Bacterial infections** from introducing bacteria deep into tissues.

- **Perforation of the rectum or colon** — a **medical emergency** that can quickly cause life-threatening infection (peritonitis) and requires urgent surgery.
- **Severe internal bleeding** from tearing large blood vessels in the rectal wall or surrounding tissues.
- **Rupture of a pre-existing aortic aneurysm** due to extreme strain during deep penetration — rare but documented in medical literature.

Think About Access to Emergency Care

A rectal perforation can lead to **sepsis within hours**. Survival and recovery depend on rapid surgery and IV antibiotics.
If you are **more than 15 minutes from a trauma center or hospital with surgical capability**, think twice about engaging in aggressive fisting or very large toy play.
The longer it takes to get emergency care, the greater the risk of serious complications or death.

Recognizing a Medical Emergency

Seek **emergency care immediately** if you or a partner experience after fisting or large toy play:

- Severe or worsening abdominal pain
- Rapid heartbeat, dizziness, or fainting
- Heavy rectal bleeding
- Fever, chills, or signs of infection
- Abdominal swelling
- Inability to pass stool or gas

Safety Guidelines

- **Start small**: Use fingers or smaller toys to gradually stretch.
- **Use plenty of thick, long-lasting lube** — silicone-based is often preferred for this type of play.
- **Communicate constantly**: Check in often about sensations.
- **Trim and file nails** completely smooth; remove rings and watches.
- **Use gloves** to reduce STI and bacterial risk (and make cleanup easier).
- **Avoid sudden force**: All stretching should be slow and deliberate.
- **Know your limits**: Extreme stretching increases tear and perforation risk.
- **Avoid playing under the influence** of drugs or alcohol that impair pain perception — pain is your body's warning system.
- **Have a plan** for what you'll do if an emergency happens — know where the nearest trauma center is.

□ PATIENT CHECKLIST – Fisting & Large Toy Safety

- ☑ Warm up with smaller toys or fingers before attempting deeper play.
- ☑ Use thick lube — reapply often.
- ☑ Wear gloves; change between partners or orifices.

- ☑ Never force past resistance — stop if there's sudden sharp pain.
- ☑ Know where the nearest trauma center is and how to get there quickly.
- ☑ If you live far from emergency surgical care, reconsider high-risk play.
- ☑ Seek immediate care if you notice signs of perforation or infection.

Watersports — Enjoyment with Awareness

Watersports, or **urine play**, can be a safe and enjoyable part of sexual expression for some people, especially when participants understand the real — and sometimes misunderstood — health risks.

How Risky Is It?

Urine from a healthy, well-hydrated person is generally low in bacteria and considered medically sterile when it leaves the bladder. However, risk increases if the person:

- Has a **urinary tract infection (UTI)**
- Has certain **sexually transmitted infections** (e.g., chlamydia, gonorrhea, trichomonas) that can live in the urethra and contaminate urine during passage
- Has **blood in the urine** (which can transmit bloodborne viruses if present)
- Has been drinking alcohol or using recreational drugs — these can irritate tissues and affect hydration

Potential Infection Risks

- **Low to moderate risk** of bacterial STIs if urine contacts mucous membranes (eyes, mouth, urethra, vagina, rectum)
- **Hepatitis B** can be present in urine of infected individuals, though transmission risk is lower than via blood or semen — hepatitis B vaccination protects against this risk
- **Hepatitis A** transmission is theoretically possible if urine is contaminated with fecal particles — vaccination is protective
- **Leptospirosis** (a rare bacterial infection) can be spread if urine from an infected person gets into mucous membranes or open cuts
- **Cytomegalovirus or CMV** can be present in urine and cause problems for people who are immunosuppressed or are on immunomodulatory medications.

Safer Watersports Practices

- Limit contact with **mucous membranes** (especially eyes and mouth) unless both partners are tested and infection-free
- Use barriers (condoms, dental dams) if playing with urine internally (e.g., into vagina or anus)
- If doing oral watersports, agree beforehand whether swallowing is on the table
- Make sure the person urinating has **no current UTI or STI symptoms**
- Hydrate well before play — clear or light yellow urine is less irritating than dark, concentrated urine

About Drinking Urine

While ingesting small amounts of urine during play are generally harmless for healthy people, **large quantities — especially if dark and concentrated — can be dangerous.** Risks include:

- **Excess salt and waste products** overloading the kidneys
- **Nausea, vomiting, or diarrhea** from high urea content
- Worsening dehydration (especially if already overheated or intoxicated)

Pro tip: Urine is not a substitute for drinking water. In fact, in survival situations, drinking urine is discouraged because it accelerates dehydration.

💧 PATIENT CHECKLIST – Watersports Safety

- ☑ Discuss boundaries — including whether contact with mouth or swallowing is okay
- ☑ Ensure both partners are up to date on hepatitis A & B vaccines
- ☑ Hydrate before play to reduce concentration and irritation

- ☑ Avoid if you have UTI symptoms, open sores, or STIs in the urethra
- ☑ Limit or avoid drinking large amounts of concentrated urine
- ☑ Use barriers if playing internally with urine

BDSM — Safe, Sane, and Consensual

BDSM encompasses a wide range of activities — bondage, discipline, dominance/submission, sadomasochism — and can be physically intense. While injury risk is low when practiced carefully, poor technique or lack of communication can cause nerve damage, blood clots, or psychological harm.

Key Risks:

- **Nerve compression** from tight restraints can cause numbness or weakness (especially wrists and ankles).
- **Circulatory problems** if restraints or cuffs cut off blood flow — this can cause clotting or tissue damage.
- **Skin injuries** (abrasions, burns, welts).
- **Emotional distress** if scenes are not negotiated or aftercare is skipped.

Safer Practices:

- Use wide, padded restraints instead of thin rope or cuffs for prolonged bondage.
- Check circulation frequently — skin should stay warm and pink.
- Avoid tying around joints or neck.

- Agree on safe words and stop immediately if they're used.
- Plan aftercare: time together after a scene to reconnect, hydrate, and check for injuries.

□ **PATIENT CHECKLIST – BDSM Safety**

- ☑ Agree on limits and safe words before starting.
- ☑ Use padded restraints and check circulation often.
- ☑ Keep scissors or a quick-release tool nearby.
- ☑ Avoid bondage around the neck or chest that restricts breathing.
- ☑ Provide aftercare and emotional check-ins post-scene.

Breath Play — Why It's Always High Risk

Breath control (erotic asphyxiation) — restricting oxygen through choking, suffocation, or airway pressure — is **inherently dangerous and potentially deadly**. It is without question a sexual fetish that is best left as a fantasy unexplored. Even brief oxygen loss can cause brain injury, sudden cardiac arrest, or death. The risks exist even when participants are careful and experienced.

Why It's Risky:

- Oxygen deprivation can cause fainting in seconds — falls may cause head injury.
- Irregular heart rhythms can occur even after oxygen is restored.
- Carotid artery pressure can trigger stroke or clot formation.

- People have died during consensual breath play even with partners present.

Harm Reduction Steps (If You Still Choose to Engage):

- Avoid any direct airway obstruction — focus only on symbolic or light touch.
- Do **not** wrap items around the neck or tie scarves/rope that could tighten unexpectedly.
- Avoid if alone — there should always be a sober, attentive partner.
- Have emergency skills and a phone ready to call EMS.

⚠ PATIENT CHECKLIST – Breath Play Risks

- ☑ Understand there is no 100% safe method — risk of death is real.
- ☑ Avoid direct airway or carotid artery compression.
- ☑ Never play alone; have a safety partner.
- ☑ Learn CPR and have EMS number ready.
- ☑ Stop immediately if dizziness or confusion occurs.

Electroplay — Shock Without Harm

Electroplay uses controlled electrical stimulation for erotic sensation. Done right, it can be safe — done wrong, it can cause burns, nerve injury, or cardiac arrest.

Safer Electroplay Basics:

- Use **only** devices designed for erotic use — avoid makeshift devices or modified electronics.
- Avoid placing electrodes on or near the chest — electrical current through the heart can be fatal.
- Keep electrodes away from broken skin to avoid burns or infections.
- Do not use if you have a pacemaker, defibrillator, or known heart rhythm problems.
- Start at the lowest intensity and increase slowly.

⚡ PATIENT CHECKLIST – Electroplay Safety

- ☑ Use commercial erotic electro-stimulation devices.
- ☑ Keep current below the waist; never across the chest or head.
- ☑ Avoid use with heart conditions or implanted devices.
- ☑ Clean and dry skin before attaching electrodes.
- ☑ Increase intensity gradually — avoid sudden jolts.

Vacuum Pumping – Pleasure Without Injury

Vacuum pumping uses negative pressure to increase blood flow to the penis or scrotum. It can enhance sensitivity, create a temporary size increase, or be part of fetish play — but overuse can cause **bruising, skin damage, or permanent vascular injury**.

Vacuum Pumping Safety

☑ Use proper equipment.

☑ Low pressure, short sessions.

☑ Remove rings within 30 minutes.
☑ Stop for pain, numbness, or color change.

Myths & Facts About Kink & Fetish Play

Myth: BDSM is always dangerous or abusive.
Fact: When practiced with clear consent, communication, and safety measures, BDSM can be as safe — or safer — than conventional sex. Abuse happens when consent is absent, not because of the activities themselves.

Myth: Only people with "issues" or past trauma are into kink.
Fact: People of all backgrounds, personalities, and histories enjoy fetish and kink play. Desire for kink is not inherently linked to past trauma.

Myth: Fisting and large toy play always cause serious injury.
Fact: While these activities have higher risk than most sexual practices, careful preparation, lube, and gradual progression can greatly reduce harm. Serious complications are rare with informed, cautious play.

Myth: Watersports can give you every STI.
Fact: Urine from healthy people carries low infection risk, but risk rises if there's a UTI, STI, or blood present. Hepatitis B vaccination offers protection against one possible infection.

Myth: Breath play can be made completely safe with experience.
Fact: No — even skilled players can't eliminate the risk of brain damage, stroke, or death. The danger comes from oxygen deprivation itself, not just inexperience.

Myth: Kink is only about pain.
Fact: Many fetishes and BDSM scenes focus on sensation, roleplay, psychological dynamics, or erotic rituals — pain is just one possible element.

🎭 PATIENT CHECKLIST – Truths About Kink

- ☑ Consent is the foundation — without it, it's abuse.
- ☑ Kink interest is normal and found in all walks of life.
- ☑ Safety measures drastically reduce (but don't remove) risks.
- ☑ Not all kink involves pain or injury.
- ☑ Some activities (like breath play) remain high-risk no matter the skill level.

Closing Thoughts

Sex practices and fetishes are part of human diversity. When approached with **enthusiastic consent, mindful hygiene, and mutual respect**, they can be deeply fulfilling and safe. This chapter isn't here to tell you what you "should" enjoy — only to give you tools so you can explore your sexuality without unnecessary health risks.

Where to Learn More & Find Safer Sex Resources

Exploring kink, fetishes, and alternative sexual practices can be exciting — and safer when you have access to the right education, community, and healthcare support. The resources below can help you **learn new skills, stay healthy, and find providers who understand your needs**.

Kink & Fetish Education

- **The National Coalition for Sexual Freedom (NCSF)** – ncsfreedom.org
  Advocates for sexual freedom and provides resources on consent, kink safety, and finding kink-aware professionals.
- **Kink Academy** – kinkacademy.com
  Subscription-based video tutorials on BDSM techniques, consent, and safety — taught by experienced educators.
- **The Eulenspiegel Society (TES)** – tes.org
  One of the oldest BDSM education and support organizations; offers classes, events, and community forums.

Safer Sex & STI Prevention

- **CDC Sexual Health** – cdc.gov/sexualhealth
  Evidence-based information on STI prevention, testing, and treatment.
- **Local LGBTQ+ Community Centers**
  Many host safer sex workshops, free testing events, and kink-friendly discussion groups.

Kink-Aware Healthcare

- **Kink Aware Professionals Directory (KAP)** – ncsfreedom.org/kap

A searchable directory of healthcare providers, therapists, and legal professionals who are kink-friendly.

- **GLMA: Health Professionals Advancing LGBTQ+ Equality** – glma.org
  Directory of LGBTQ+-competent healthcare providers across specialties.

Consent & Sexual Rights Advocacy

- **Consent Academy** – consent.academy
  Workshops and resources on consent skills for sexual and nonsexual contexts.
- **Scarleteen** – scarleteen.com
  Inclusive sex education site with sections on kink, boundaries, and communication.

Workshops & Events

- **Munches** – Informal meetups for kink enthusiasts, usually held in public spaces like cafes or restaurants. Great for meeting the local community in a non-sexual setting.
  Search: "[Your City] Munch" on FetLife or Meetup.
- **FetLife** – fetlife.com
  Social networking platform for kink communities; events, discussions, and local group listings.

☐ PATIENT CHECKLIST – Finding Safer Sex Resources

- ☑ Learn from credible, experienced educators.
- ☑ Verify your healthcare provider is kink-aware before sharing details.
- ☑ Stay updated on STI prevention and testing.
- ☑ Connect with local kink-friendly communities for peer support.
- ☑ Attend workshops to build skill and confidence.

Chapter 11 – Anal Care: Douching, Toys, Fisting & Trauma Prevention

When I first started writing the Tom of P-Town Health blog on Bluesky, I never guessed which post would take off the most. But to this day, the **most-read article of all them all** is the one on anal douching. That shows something important: people want real, trustworthy information on anal care—but it's still surprisingly hard to find.

I'll admit something personal here: for years, I didn't bottom at all. Not because I didn't want to, but because the stress of cleaning out was overwhelming. No one ever explained how you were "supposed" to do it. Was it safe? Was it bad for your health? Were you even *meant* to do it at all? And worst of all…. What if you didn't do it well enough? How could you know? What if there was a unwelcome surprise? The resources were practically nonexistent, and it's still not something we really talk about.

Thirty years later, it's still tough to find good, clear guidance. People often end up learning from porn, word of mouth, or trial and error—which is hardly a recipe for feeling confident in your body.

And here's another truth: in medicine, the rectum is **not thought of as a sexual organ**. For providers who aren't LGBTQ themselves—or who haven't taken the time to learn—this leads to a serious lack of appreciation for how much the rectum matters to their patients' sexual lives and overall wellbeing. Disfigurement, infection, damage, or scarring aren't just "complications"—they can take away pleasure, intimacy, and even a piece of identity. Even if you have an LGBTQ-informed primary care provider, at some point you'll likely see a specialist who doesn't see the rectum through this lens. And when that happens, your needs may be dismissed or misunderstood. For example, a colostomy is a huge deal for everyone- but for a gay man it has implications far beyond those a straight person faces.

This gap in knowledge is especially important when it comes to practices like **fisting**. While for many it can be deeply erotic and affirming, the risks are real. Over my career, as I shared in the previous chapter, I've seen what can happen when those risks turn into tragedy. That doesn't mean the answer is fear—it means the answer is *knowledge*. Understanding how to care for the rectum, how to prepare for play, and where the limits are can make the difference between a safe, pleasurable experience and a medical emergency.

That's the reason behind this chapter: To show you what safe, practical anal care looks like—not just douching, but preparation, healing, and included some reflection on practices that carry risk. To help you feel clean, comfortable, confident, and empowered in your choices.

Because everyone deserves to **discover their inner bottom** without fear, shame, or confusion.

Your butt is more than just an erogenous zone — it's a delicate and amazing part of your body that deserves respect, care, and attention. Whether you're exploring anal play for the first time or you're a seasoned pro, knowing how to protect your health and avoid injury will help you enjoy it for years to come.

1 | Understanding the Anatomy

The rectum and anus contain sensitive nerve endings, muscles, and a mucosal lining that is *not* designed to take heavy friction or trauma. There's no natural lubrication here — so lube and gentleness are essential.

Key points:

- **Sphincter muscles** control opening and closing — forcing them open can cause tears.
- **Rectal lining** is thin and fragile compared to vaginal tissue — easier to injure.
- **Blood supply** means injuries can bleed a lot, and bacteria can enter the bloodstream.

2 | Douching — How to Do It Safely

Many people douche before receptive anal play to feel clean, but overdoing it can irritate the lining and increase STI risk. A safe routine depends on two things:

1. **The apparatus** — what you use to deliver the liquid
2. **The solution** — what liquid you put into it

A. Apparatus Options

Apparatus	Description	Benefits	Risks/Misc
Reusable bulb (many brands)	Hand-squeezed silicone or rubber bulb with removable nozzle	Affordable over time; good control of volume; compatible with different solutions	Must be cleaned thoroughly after each use; not sterile
Future Method bulb	Premium silicone bulb designed for anal use	High quality; easy to clean; pairs with their pH-balanced solution	Higher cost; still requires cleaning
Gravity-fed enema bag	Bag with tubing/nozzle that relies on gravity	Allows more gradual flow; easy volume control	Bulkier; requires more setup; tubing must be cleaned well
Shower enema attachments	Nozzle/tubing that connects to a shower hose for continuous water flow	No refilling needed; adjustable flow via shower controls	**High injury risk** from excessive pressure; can over-flush and strip protective lining; must be used at *very* low

Apparatus	Description	Benefits	Risks/Misc
			flow and safe temperature
Pre-filled disposable enema bottle	Single-use bottle with built-in nozzle	Convenient; portable; no cleaning needed	More waste; ongoing cost; often contains harsh solutions

B. Solution Options

Solution	Benefits	Risks/Considerations
Future Method cleansing solution	Pre-mixed, isotonic, pH-balanced to reduce irritation	Higher cost; single-use bottles create more packaging waste
Homemade isotonic saline(e.g., with NeilMed kit)	Gentle on rectal lining; inexpensive; can be used in reusable bulbs	Requires correct salt measurement; mild prep time
Plain tap water	Cheap; readily available	Temperature extremes or chlorine may cause irritation; less gentle than saline
Fleet® enemas (phosphate-based)	Very effective at clearing quickly	Can cause cramping, irritation, or electrolyte imbalance; avoid frequent use

General Douching Safety Tips

- **Water temperature**: Lukewarm (body temp) — test on inner wrist.
- **Volume**: 1–2 bulb fills or equivalent is usually enough if you use isotonic solution.
- **Technique**:
    1. Lube the nozzle generously.
    2. Insert gently (≤2 inches).
    3. Squeeze or allow fluid to flow slowly.
    4. Hold briefly, then release into the toilet.
- **Avoid high pressure** — especially with shower attachments; keep flow low to prevent injury.
- **Timing**: Finish at least 30–60 minutes before play.

Special Notes — Anal Fissures & Hemorrhoids

- **Anal fissures**: Painful small tears in the lining, aggravated by trauma or constipation.
- **Hemorrhoids**: Swollen veins that may itch, bleed, or be tender.
- **Seek medical attention** if:
    - Bleeding is heavy or persistent
    - Severe pain or swelling occurs
    - Fever, pus, or signs of infection appear
    - There's suspected deep tear or perforation

Avoid douching during active flare-ups to prevent worsening the condition.

3 | Toys — Size, Shape & Safety

Sex toys can be a great addition to anal play — but not all toys are created equal.

Safety checklist:

- **Flared base or retrieval cord** — prevents the dreaded "trip to the ER" for a lost toy.
- **Body-safe materials** — silicone, stainless steel, and glass are safest; avoid porous plastics that trap bacteria.
- **Start small, build up** — rushing to larger sizes risks tearing and muscle strain.
- **Clean thoroughly** — warm water + mild soap after every use; boil silicone or stainless steel toys if safe for the material.
- **Use plenty of lube** — and reapply often. Silicone lube lasts longer, water-based lube is easier to wash off.

4 | Fisting & Large-Toy Play — Proceed with Care

Fisting and extra-large toys can be pleasurable but carry real risks, including:

- Deep tears in the rectum
- Damage to the sphincter muscles which can result in incontinence and prolapse "Rosebuds" are being fetishized online but in real life having rectal prolapse can lead to incontinence, tissue strangulation and necrosis that necessitates surgery or even colostomy and significant liquid discharge that requires diaper wearing.

- Damage to the **pudendal and pelvic splanchnic nerves** which can
- **Rare but life-threatening complications** like **perforation** (a hole in the rectum/colon) or rupture of nearby blood vessels, including the aorta can and have happened.
- **If you're more than 15 minutes from a trauma center**, think twice — a perforation can quickly lead to sepsis (life threatening infection) and requires immediate high-level emergency care especially if you're a newbie- wait till you back home in the big city for your first time.

Safer fisting guidelines:

- **Consent and communication** — both partners must be on the same page.
- **Warm-up** — start with fingers, then more, then slowly progress.
- **Relaxation is key** — rushing is the #1 cause of injury.
- **Copious lube** — use more than you think you need.
- **Know the signs of trouble** — sudden severe pain, bleeding, fever, or abdominal swelling = ER now.

5 | Trauma Prevention & Aftercare

Even with care, small tears or irritation can happen. Here's how to minimize damage:

- **Stop immediately** if there's sharp pain.

- **Avoid alcohol or heavy drugs** before intense play — they dull pain warning signs.
- **Give your body time to recover** — take a break if you've had significant stretching or bruising.
- **Aftercare** — rinse gently, apply a water-based barrier gel to external areas if irritated, seek help if significant or ongoing bleeding and monitor for signs of infection (redness, pus, swelling, fever).

6 | Sexual Health & Testing

Anal play can increase your risk for certain STIs, including gonorrhea, chlamydia, HPV, and herpes. Protect yourself by:

- **Consider using condoms** for anal intercourse
- **Getting screened every 3 months** if you're sexually active with multiple partners
- **Vaccinating** for HPV and hepatitis A & B

7 | Bottom Line

Anal play can be intensely pleasurable and deeply intimate. With preparation, respect for your body, and open communication with your partners, you can enjoy it safely. Treat your butt well — it's the only one you've got.

Patient Exercise:
List your current anal play practices (type, frequency, toys used, douching habits). Identify one change you could make to reduce irritation or injury risk while keeping pleasure high.

Some suggestions and thoughts about Fisting, Intimacy, and Self-Reflection

Fisting is a sexual practice that, while rare compared to other activities is growing in popularity, it can be deeply intense—physically and emotionally. For some, it's about pushing physical boundaries; for others, it can feel like a profoundly intimate connection. This section invites you to pause, reflect, and explore your motivations, while also understanding the possible risks. It's important to consider there may be safer ways to meet the need that's driving your interest. At Tom of P-Town we are sex positive and don't judge but as I've shared I've had patients die getting fisted and tops that had to worry about facing possible manslaughter charges so the current culture of treating it as a common activity that can be done roughly gives me a lot of concern. Go through our reflection or use the understanding your motivation worksheet below to help navigate your underlying motivations and make informed decisions.

1. Reflecting on Motivation

Ask yourself:

- **What draws me to fisting?**
  Is it the thrill of physical sensation, the trust required, the taboo nature, or a mix of these?
- **Am I seeking a deeper connection?**
  Sometimes, the desire for intense physical closeness masks a deeper craving for emotional intimacy, vulnerability, or being "fully known" by a partner.

- **Does this fit into my overall sexual wellness?** Consider whether the practice supports your physical, emotional, and relational health.

Exercise:
Write down three words that describe what you hope to feel during or after fisting. Then ask:

- Could I get these feelings in other, safer ways?
- Would I still want this if those feelings were met elsewhere in my life?

2. Risks and Realities

While fatalities are **rare**, they **do happen**—usually from internal tears, perforations, or severe trauma. Even without an emergency, long-term effects can include:

- Chronic changes in anal sphincter tone
- Loss of fine muscle control
- Increased risk for hemorrhoids or prolapse

These are not guaranteed outcomes, but they are possibilities worth weighing honestly.

Reality check:
Would this practice still be appealing if it carried a permanent physical change you didn't expect?

3. Discerning Intimacy

If intimacy is the draw, think about other ways to meet that need:

- Extended skin-to-skin contact
- Eye contact and slower, sustained touch

- Erotic massage
- Shared vulnerability through conversation or roleplay

Exercise:
Try a "nonpenetrative intimacy session" with your partner where the goal is connection, not climax. Afterwards, compare how you feel with how you typically feel after more intense play. This can help clarify whether fisting is about the physical act itself or the emotional state it produces.

Key takeaway:
Fisting can be a meaningful part of sexual expression for some people, but it's worth ensuring that the choice is driven by your authentic desires—not by an unmet emotional need that could be met more safely. By reflecting first, you can approach the practice with both self-awareness and informed caution.

Fisting & Intimacy Self-Reflection Worksheet

This worksheet is for personal use only. You don't need to share your answers with anyone unless you choose to.
Be honest with yourself — there are no right or wrong responses.

Part 1 — Understanding Your Motivation

1. **What draws me to the idea of fisting?**
   (Check all that apply)
   ☐ Physical intensity or challenge
   ☐ Emotional closeness / trust
   ☐ Taboo or novelty
   ☐ Desire to please a partner

☐ Curiosity / exploration

☐ Other: ____________________________

2. **Describe in your own words what you hope to feel during or after the experience:**

3. **If I could get these feelings in a different, safer way, would I still want to try fisting?**

   ☐ Yes

   ☐ No

   ☐ Not sure — I'd like to explore further

Part 2 — A Reality Check

4. **What risks am I aware of?**
   (Check all that apply)

   ☐ Anal tears or injury

   ☐ Perforation (life-threatening emergency)

   ☐ Infection risk

   ☐ Long-term changes in sphincter tone or muscle control

   ☐ Hemorrhoids or prolapse

   ☐ Emotional impact / regret

5. **How would I feel if this caused a permanent change to my body?**

Part 3 — Exploring the Intimacy Factor

6. **When I imagine fisting, do I picture more of…**
   ☐ The physical act itself
   ☐ The emotional closeness it creates
   ☐ Both equally
7. **Other ways I might meet my intimacy needs:**
   ☐ Extended skin-to-skin contact
   ☐ Eye contact and slow, sustained touch
   ☐ Erotic massage
   ☐ Shared vulnerability through conversation or roleplay
   ☐ Other: ______________________________
8. **Plan an "intimacy-only" session with a partner** (no penetration). Afterward, write how you felt compared to what you expected:

Part 4 — My Decision

9. **After reflection, my feelings about fisting are:**
   ☐ I feel informed and still want to try, with precautions
   ☐ I want to wait and explore my intimacy needs first
   ☐ I've decided it's not right for me at this time

Reminder:
Fisting can be meaningful for some people, but it carries real risks. If you choose to explore it, communicate openly with partners, go slowly, and use plenty of lubrication. Know the signs of injury, and seek medical help if needed and be ready to deal with health complications if they arise.

Chapter 12

Group & Party Sex: Risk-Reduction Moves That Actually Work

Group & Party Sex: Risk-Reduction Moves That Actually Work

In more than twenty-two years of caring for gay, bisexual, and other men who have sex with men, one of the hardest truths I've had to face—and witness over and over—is how often sexual assault occurs, and how rarely it's named for what it is: rape. Too many of my patients, and even some of my friends, have endured these experiences without ever using that word, as though the absence of language could blunt the trauma.

I'll never forget a date I went on with a guy who shared with me that his previous boyfriend drugged him and left him in an outdoor sling at a gay resort in Palm Springs; he came to with a stranger inside him and a line of others waiting their turn. Or a patient who described a threesome with his boyfriend and a third man that turned violent when the guest double penetrated him while he was engaged with his boyfriend from behind without consent, tearing his external sphincter and leaving him in need of surgery. Still another patient shared that he trusted a date enough to take them home—only to be physically held down and raped. These are not misunderstandings, they are not "gray zones," and they are not erased by whatever drugs or consensual acts might have come before. If you have not given consent, it is rape. And if you engage someone who has not consented, you have committed rape. Period.

That clarity matters, because the stakes are high. Rape causes real trauma—physical, psychological, and relational—and I've seen the damage firsthand. So before we talk about safer group sex practices, here's what I want you to carry with you:

- **Do not compromise your ability to consent.** If drugs or alcohol are in play, know your limits.
- **Establish or verify consent monitors.** In a group or party setting, someone needs to keep an eye on dynamics and step in if consent is violated if there is no such person find another group.
- **Respect boundaries, every time.** No matter how heated things get, stop if someone says "no" or doesn't say "yes."
- **Report perpetrators.** If someone rapes you, know that reporting them is not just about your own healing—it protects others who may not have your strength or voice.

Group and party sex can be fun, affirming, and even healing when handled with care. But without clear consent and respect, it can cause lasting harm. In this chapter we'll look at risk-reduction strategies—covering not only STI prevention and safer substance use, but also how to navigate consent, boundaries, and respect in group sexual spaces.

Group and party sex can be exciting, liberating, and deeply satisfying. It can also carry unique physical and emotional risks. This chapter isn't here to judge your choices — it's here to give you tools so you can enjoy yourself while protecting your health and your partners.

Understanding the Risks

In group settings, you're potentially exposed to:

- **More partners in a short time** → higher chance of sexually transmitted infections (STIs)
- **Mixing of body fluids** (semen, saliva, lubricant) between multiple people
- **Breaks in skin or mucosa** from friction, fisting, toys, or vigorous activity
- **Drug and alcohol use** affecting judgment and safer sex practices
- **Reduced clarity on consent** if boundaries aren't talked about beforehand

Risk-Reduction Moves That Actually Work

1. Plan Before You Play

- Decide ahead of time what activities you're open to and what's off the table stick to it.
- If possible agree on boundaries with partners before you engage — it's much easier than negotiating mid-play.

Pro tip:
Suggest the organizers have a universal "safe word" or "time-out" gesture in case you or others need to stop.

2. Consider Using Barriers

- **Consider condoms** for anal or oral sex can reduce risk of HIV and many STIs.
  If condoms aren't your choice, make sure you're on HIV prevention (PrEP or undetectable if living with HIV) and get frequent STI testing.

- **Consider gloves** for fisting or toy sharing — change gloves or wash hands between partners.
- **Consider dental dams** for oral-anal contact.

3. Lube Wisely

- Use *lots* of lube — it reduces tears, friction, and discomfort.
- Water-based or silicone-based lubes are best for condoms and gloves.
- Avoid oil-based lubes with latex — they can weaken it.

4. Change or Clean Between Partners

- If using barriers swap your condoms, gloves, and toy covers before moving to another partner.
- Wipe down toys with disinfectant wipes or wash with soap and water.
- Don't share douching equipment! Hep C is hard to kill and can be spread this way.

5. Be Smart About Substances

- Alcohol and drugs can make it harder to stick to boundaries or recognize signs of injury.
- If you choose to use, plan your limits ahead of time and have a trusted friend keep an eye out for you.

6. Mind the Physical Risks

- Aggressive fisting or large toy play can cause serious injuries, including tears or perforations which can result in death.
  If you're more than 15 minutes from a trauma center, think twice and be extra careful— perforations can be life-threatening.
- Heavy anal play increases the chance of hemorrhoids, fissures, and pelvic floor strain.

7. Keep an Eye on Consent

- Consent can fade if someone becomes impaired or overwhelmed.
- Check in with partners regularly — a simple "You good?" can go a long way.

After the Party

- **Shower and clean up** — reduces skin irritation and helps you check for injuries.
- **STI testing**: Many sexually active men who have sex with men benefit from testing every 3 months, but after a high-exposure event, sooner can be better.
- **Treat injuries promptly** — even small tears can get infected.
- **Emotional check-in**: After intense group play, some people feel a "drop" in mood. This is normal. Reach out to friends or partners for support.

Exercise — Your Risk-Reduction Game Plan

Before your next group or party event:

1. List your **yes**, **no**, and **maybe** activities.
2. Decide on your barrier use plan if you will be using one or more (condoms, consider gloves, toy cleaning).
3. Arrange your testing schedule before and after.
4. Pack your "party kit":
    - Consider Condoms
    - Lube
    - Consider gloves
    - Toy covers
    - Disinfectant wipes
    - Water and snacks
    - A discreet bag for used barriers

Bottom line:
Group sex can be part of a healthy, fulfilling sex life if approached with preparation, respect, and care. The more you plan, the more you can relax and enjoy yourself — without letting risks ruin the fun.

Chapter 13

Beyond the Basics: Sounding, Pumps, Breath Play & Other Edge Activities

Let's make no mistake up front: **Tom of P-Town Health does not recommend sounding or breath play.** Both are high-risk practices, and in the case of breath play the danger is often fatal. In fact, with breath play death is not an uncommon outcome—it is a tragically predictable one. The "benefits" people describe—heightened sensation, trust, or intimacy—can almost always be achieved through **safer activities** that do not carry the same life-altering or life-ending consequences.

So why include these practices in this chapter at all? Because in more than two decades of caring for gay, bisexual, and queer men, I've learned that discouragement alone doesn't stop people. Some of you are going to do it anyway. And if you do, I would much rather you have **accurate information** that can at least reduce some of the harm. **But let me be clear: making something *safer* is not the same as making it *safe*. Just like condoms are used for safer sex, all sex has some risk, it is not safe.**

- **Sounding** (the insertion of objects into the urethra) carries significant risks of infection, urethral trauma, and long-term complications like strictures or loss of sexual function.
- **Breath play** (restricting oxygen for sexual arousal) is unpredictable, unforgiving, and has directly resulted in countless deaths—even among people who were experienced, healthy, and careful.

In this chapter, I'll outline what these practices involve, why they are so dangerous, and—if you choose to proceed against medical advice—what steps can at least lower some of the risks. My hope is that by being honest, we can preserve health, prevent trauma, and maybe even dissuade some from pursuing activities where the cost is far too high. Other activities in this chapter like wax and electroplay have risks as well but if some care is used, they are rarely fatal or crippling so have at it but read up and educate yourself first.

Some sexual practices push the body — and sometimes the mind — beyond what most people consider "typical."
These "edge activities" can create intense sensations, taboo excitement, and feelings of trust or control.
They also carry higher risks — sometimes life-threatening ones.
Here's how to approach them with **eyes open and safety first**.

Sounding (Urethral Play)

What it is:
Inserting a smooth rod, catheter, or toy into the urethra — the tube that carries urine and semen.

Why people do it:

- Unique, deep sensations from stimulating nerve endings inside the urethra and prostate
- Erotic taboo — "doing something forbidden" can be arousing
- Roleplay or medical kink
- Trust and power exchange

Risks:

- **Infection:** UTIs or bladder infections from introducing bacteria directly into the urinary tract
- **Tears and bleeding** from forcing a sound or using rough/unsafe objects
- **Urethral strictures** — scar tissue that narrows the urethra and can require surgery
- **Internal organ injury:** Inserting too deeply can pass beyond the bladder into the ureters or toward the prostate and surrounding structures, risking injury to the bladder wall or even internal bleeding — this is a **medical emergency**

Equipment & safe practice:

- Use **medical-grade stainless steel sounds** or sterile, single-use catheters
- Avoid chrome-plated, aluminum, or poor-quality metal — coatings can flake into tissue
- Choose a slightly tapered, rounded tip — not pointed or sharp
- **Sterilization:** Autoclave if possible; if not, boil metal for at least 10 minutes, remove with sterile tongs, and cool in a clean container
- Wash hands and genitals thoroughly, and use sterile gloves if possible
- Only use **sterile, water-based lubricant** in single-use packets
- Insert slowly, never force — if you feel pain or resistance, stop immediately
- Beginners should **never insert beyond the base of the penis** — deeper insertion greatly increases the risk of bladder or organ injury

Pumps (Penis or Scrotum Pumping)

What it is:
A device that creates a vacuum to draw blood into the penis or scrotum for temporary enlargement.

Why people do it:

- Increased erection firmness
- Temporary size boost for visual or performance purposes
- Sensation of suction and stretch
- Part of BDSM or humiliation play

Risks:

- Bruising, blisters, or broken blood vessels
- Numbness or nerve injury from overpressure
- Long-term skin looseness or discoloration from chronic overuse

Equipment & safe practice:

- **Always use a pump designed for erections** — not homemade devices, brake bleeder kits, or vacuum cleaners
- **Cylinder:** Clear acrylic lets you see skin color and swelling
- **Seal:** Soft silicone or rubber base for comfort
- **Pressure control:** Must have a built-in gauge — stay under 5 inHg for beginners
- **Manual hand pumps** allow more control than cheap electric pumps
- Avoid devices without a quick-release valve — they can trap dangerous vacuum pressure
- Start with short sessions (5–10 minutes), slowly building up to a max of 15–20 minutes

- If skin becomes cold, pale, or blue — **release immediately**
- Clean after each use with warm soapy water, rinse, and air dry

Breath Play (Erotic Asphyxiation)

What it is:
Restricting airflow or blood flow to the brain to heighten sexual sensation.

Why people do it:

- Perceived intensification of orgasm from oxygen deprivation
- Power and vulnerability exchange
- Adrenaline rush from the risk

Why we **strongly recommend against it:

- Even experienced participants have died — the **fatality rate is significant**, and incidents happen quickly, often within seconds
- Brain damage can occur in under 4 minutes without oxygen
- There is no fully "safe" technique — many deaths happen even when partners are present and attentive
- Solo breath play is particularly deadly, as there's no one to intervene if you lose consciousness

If you still choose to proceed despite the risks:

- Never play alone — always have a sober, attentive partner

- Avoid compressing the front of the neck — if restricting blood flow, keep sessions extremely short
- Use verbal and physical check-ins — but know they may fail if someone passes out
- Have a rapid-release plan and know basic CPR

Electro-Play

What it is:
Using controlled electrical current to stimulate nerves, muscles, or skin during sexual activity.

Why people do it:

- Tingling, buzzing, and deep muscle contraction sensations
- Heightened arousal from nerve stimulation
- Aesthetic and psychological appeal — "sci-fi," "medical," or "control" play themes

Risks:

- Burns or skin irritation from poor contact
- Involuntary muscle contractions that may cause injury
- Dangerous heart rhythm changes if current passes through the chest — potentially fatal for those with heart conditions or implanted devices
- Risk of nerve injury with prolonged or intense exposure

Equipment & safe practice:

- **Only use devices made for erotic or medical use** (TENS units, violet wands, or commercial electrosex machines) — **never jury-rig from household electronics**

- Electrodes should be placed on fleshy areas — **never across the chest or head**
- Use conductive gel to reduce hot spots and burns
- Start at the lowest setting and increase slowly
- Inspect wires and electrodes for damage before use
- Clean skin contact points before and after play to reduce irritation and infection risk

Wax Play (Low-Temperature Wax)

What it is:
Dripping warm wax on the skin for sensation play.

Why people do it:

- Sensory contrast — heat followed by cooling
- Ritualistic or artistic appeal in kink scenes

Risks:

- Burns if wax is too hot
- Allergic reactions to dyes or fragrances

Equipment & safe practice:

- Use low-temperature "play" or soy-based wax — **not paraffin or beeswax** from household candles
- Test temperature on the inside of your wrist before dripping on a partner
- **Avoid the face and eyes**
- Place a drop cloth to protect floors and furniture
- Clean skin after to remove residue and reduce irritation

Emotional Considerations

Edge play can involve intense trust and emotional vulnerability.

- Discuss expectations and boundaries beforehand
- Plan aftercare — cuddling, quiet time, hydration, reassurance
- Be aware of "drop" — temporary sadness, fatigue, or anxiety after intense play

Exercise — Your Edge Play Safety Plan

Before trying an edge activity:

1. **Motivation:** Why am I drawn to this? Sensation? Taboo? Connection?
2. **Preparation:** Do I have the right equipment, knowledge, and hygiene supplies?
3. **Partner choice:** Are they sober, experienced, and trustworthy?
4. **Safety plan:** What's my stop signal? What's my emergency plan?
5. **Aftercare:** What will help me feel grounded and safe afterward?

Bottom line:
These activities can bring unique sensations and experiences, but some — especially **breath play** — carry extreme dangers that can't be fully eliminated. Make your choices informed,

deliberate, and with your safety and your partner's safety at the center of the experience.

Edge Play Equipment & Cleaning Guide

Activity	Recommended Equipment	Avoid	Cleaning / Sterilization	Key Safety Checks
Sounding (Urethral Play)	Medical-grade stainless steel sounds or sterile, single-use catheters; sterile water-based lube in single-use packets; sterile gloves	Household objects, glass, coated or flaking metal, chrome-plated rods, rough or sharp tips	Autoclave if possible; boil for 10 min and cool in sterile container; wash hands before handling; store in clean sealed container	Never force; stop at pain/resistance; beginners stay shallow to avoid bladder/organ injury

Activity	Recommended Equipment	Avoid	Cleaning / Sterilization	Key Safety Checks
Pumping (Penis/Scrotum)	Clear acrylic cylinder; soft silicone/rubber base; manual hand pump with built-in pressure gauge and quick-release valve	Homemade pumps, brake bleeder kits, vacuum cleaners, electric pumps without gauge	Wash cylinder/base with warm soapy water after each use; rinse, air dry; store in clean, dry place	Keep under 5 inHg (beginners); max 15–20 min sessions; release if skin turns cold, pale, or blue
Breath Play	— *(Not recommended due to high fatality risk)* —	All forms, especially solo play, restrictive hoods, plastic bags, neck compression	— N/A —	**Strongly discouraged**: high risk of brain damage or death, even with experience and

Activity	Recommended Equipment	Avoid	Cleaning / Sterilization	Key Safety Checks
				partners present
Electro-Play	Commercial erotic electro devices (TENS units, violet wands, electrosex machines) with intact cords and electrodes; conductive gel	Household electronics, damaged cords, electrodes over heart/head	Wipe electrodes with alcohol pad after each use; check device for fraying or cracks; store dry	Avoid chest/head; start at lowest setting; increase slowly; check skin for burns or irritation
Wax Play	Low-temp "play" wax or soy candles; drop cloth; safe pour/drip tools	Paraffin/beeswax household candles; scented/dyed candles that irritate skin	Clean skin with mild soap after play; protect floors/furniture	Test wax temp on wrist; avoid face/eyes; drip slowly;

Activity	Recommended Equipment	Avoid	Cleaning / Sterilization	Key Safety Checks
				monitor skin for redness or blistering

How to Use This Table:

- **Recommended Equipment** = safest starting point
- **Avoid** = highest risk for injury or infection
- **Cleaning / Sterilization** = minimum hygiene steps every time
- **Key Safety Checks** = what to confirm before and during play

Chapter 14

Party Drugs & Chemsex: Safer-Use Checklists for Meth, GHB, Poppers, Mephedrone & More

Sex is one of life's absolute joys. It is not just a pastime—it's a biological drive, wired into our brains and bodies through millions of years of evolution. Our survival as a species depended on it, and so nature made sure we would not only do it, but want to do it often. At its best, sex is discovery: learning what excites you, how to connect with others, and how to give and receive pleasure more deeply over time.

That's why it's worth pausing before turning to chemicals to change how sex feels. Using artificial methods to enhance sexual experience isn't necessary—and it can block you from the path of discovery that lets you grow into better sex, better intimacy, and better connection. Altering your brain chemistry for a temporary high can rob you of the long-term satisfaction of building skill, confidence, and trust in your sexual life.

That said, some men do make the decision to mix drugs and sex. If you're considering it, I ask you to think carefully about whether it's truly necessary. And if you decide it is, please hear this: **Tom of P-Town Health asks all gay men never to touch crystal meth.** It is the single most destructive drug our community has ever known. And while GHB is often viewed as "fun" or "harmless," it, too, demands extreme caution—its margin of safety is razor thin, and the line between a euphoric dose and a life-threatening overdose is frighteningly small.

In this chapter, we'll walk through what chemsex means, the drugs most often involved, the risks unique to each, and harm-reduction strategies. But above all, remember: the most powerful, transformative sex you can have doesn't come from a substance—it comes from you.

Chemsex — combining sex with certain drugs to enhance pleasure, intimacy, or stamina — can be intensely rewarding but also risky.

This chapter is about *reducing harm*, *checking substances for adulteration*, and *knowing where to get help if use becomes a problem.*

Methamphetamine ("Meth," "Tina," "Crystal")

Why people use it in sex:

- Heightened arousal, euphoria, and sexual stamina
- Lowered inhibitions, increased confidence
- Prolonged sex sessions, sometimes lasting days

Why meth is uniquely dangerous:
Meth **damages the brain's self-regulation circuits**, making it extremely hard to control use.

- For some, addiction takes hold after just a few uses
- The point at which someone shifts from "recreational" to compulsive use is unpredictable
- **Because brain changes may be permanent, there is no "safe" amount or frequency of meth use**

Risks:

- Rapid heart rate, high blood pressure, overheating
- Paranoia, hallucinations, aggression
- Skin sores, dental decay
- High risk of dependence and crash depression
- Prolonged sex increases injury and STI risk

Safer-use checklist:

- Use the **smallest possible dose**; avoid "re-dosing"
- Hydrate with water/electrolytes (not excess)
- Take rest breaks to cool down
- If injecting: always use **new, sterile needles**, rotate sites, never share
- Plan food, rest, and support for the comedown

Drug testing:

- Adulterants include fentanyl, other stimulants, cutting powders
- **Fentanyl test strips** (BTNX, DanceSafe, Bunk Police)
- **Marquis or Mandelin reagents** for meth detection

Mephedrone (4-MMC, "Meph," "MCAT," "Drone")

Why people use it in sex:

- Combination of stimulant (like cocaine) and empathogen (like MDMA)
- Heightened sociability and arousal
- Prolonged sex, feelings of closeness and connection

Risks:

- Fast heart rate, high blood pressure, overheating
- Anxiety, paranoia, agitation with binges
- Nose damage (if snorted), vein and skin damage (if injected)
- Compulsive "re-dosing" every 1–2 hours → high crash risk
- Sleep deprivation and psychosis after long sessions

Safer-use checklist:

- Start small, wait before re-dosing — effects fade fast but tolerance builds quickly
- Hydrate, eat, and sleep when possible
- If snorting: use personal straw, rinse nose with saline after
- If injecting: sterile supplies only, rotate sites, never share
- Avoid marathon sessions without breaks

Drug testing:

- Frequently adulterated with other synthetic cathinones ("bath salts"), amphetamines
- **Marquis reagent**: yellow/green
- **Mecke reagent**: dark green
- Kits: **DanceSafe**, **Bunk Police**
- Full mail-in lab analysis: **Energy Control (Spain)**

GHB / GBL ("G," "Liquid Ecstasy")

Why people use it in sex:

- Euphoric, disinhibiting

- Enhanced touch sensitivity
- Bonding or "chem-intimacy" effect

Risks:

- Very narrow safe-to-toxic dose range
- Overdose: unconsciousness, slowed breathing, vomiting, death
- Mixing with alcohol or depressants is especially lethal
- Severe withdrawal if used daily

Safer-use checklist:

- Measure doses with syringe/pipette (never "cap" dosing)
- Wait **2+ hours** before re-dosing
- Never mix with alcohol, benzos, opioids
- Only use with partners who know recovery position + when to call 911
- If unconscious: **call for help — do not "let them sleep it off"**

Drug testing:

- No reliable home test; best practice is careful dosing and trusted source
- Some advanced testing via **Energy Control** (Spain)

Poppers (Amyl, Butyl, Isobutyl Nitrite)

Why people use it in sex:

- Relax anal sphincter → easier penetration
- Short-lived head rush

- Enhanced orgasm

Risks:

- Dangerous with ED meds (Viagra, Cialis, Levitra) — can cause fatal blood pressure crash
- Dizziness, fainting, headaches
- Irritation to nose, eyes, and skin

Safer-use checklist:

- Inhale vapor only; never swallow
- Avoid mixing with ED or blood pressure meds
- Store tightly sealed; bottles leak easily

Drug testing:

- Adulteration less common but mislabeling is frequent
- No home test kits available; buy only from trusted vendors

Cocaine / Crack Cocaine

Why people use it in sex:

- Increased energy, stamina, and talkativeness
- Delayed ejaculation for some
- Heightened arousal

Risks:

- Heart strain → risk of heart attack or stroke
- Paranoia, anxiety

- Nasal damage from snorting, burns from crack smoking
- High addiction risk

Safer-use checklist:

- Avoid mixing with alcohol → forms toxic **cocaethylene**
- Use your own straw/surface — avoid sharing (HCV risk)
- Stay hydrated and rest

Drug testing:

- Cocaine is often adulterated with **levamisole**, fentanyl, stimulants
- **Fentanyl test strips** are essential
- Reagent kits: **Marquis, Mecke, Scott's** (DanceSafe, Bunk Police)

Ketamine ("K")

Why people use it in sex:

- Dream-like dissociation
- Reduced pain sensitivity
- Intense, sometimes spiritual experiences

Risks:

- Impaired coordination → falls, injuries
- Amnesia → unsafe consent situations
- Long-term use → bladder/urinary tract damage ("K bladder")

- Psychological dependence possible

Safer-use checklist:

- Start small; high doses risk "K-hole" (loss of body control)
- Avoid mixing with alcohol or sedatives
- Use in safe space, ideally with sober supervision
- Stay hydrated

Drug testing:

- Ketamine often cut with stimulants or other powders
- **Mandelin reagent** best for ketamine testing (DanceSafe, Bunk Police)

One of the most important—and too often overlooked—steps in harm reduction is **testing recreational drugs for adulterants**. Street drugs are rarely pure; powders, pills, and liquids are frequently cut with other stimulants, opioids like fentanyl, or even toxic chemicals that can dramatically increase the risk of overdose, psychosis, or organ damage. Simple reagent kits, fentanyl test strips, and newer combination panels are widely available in the U.S. through harm-reduction groups and online vendors, and they can quickly identify many common adulterants. Testing doesn't make drug use safe, but it does make it **safer**, giving you information to make better choices, avoid unexpected reactions, and reduce the risk of serious harm or death. The following are some **General Testing Resources**

- **DanceSafe (dancesafe.org):** US nonprofit, sells reagent kits, fentanyl strips
- **Bunk Police (bunkpolice.com):** International reagent kit vendor

- **Energy Control (energycontrol-international.org):** Spain-based mail-in lab testing service
- **Local harm reduction centers:** Often distribute test kits, fentanyl strips, sterile supplies

Not-for-Profit & Harm Reduction Providers

- **DanceSafe**
    - A leading nonprofit that produces reagent and fentanyl/xylazine test kits for harm reduction purposes. They set industry standards in North America. arrowheadforensics.com+12DanceSafe+12Addiction Services and Supports+12
    - Their online shop also offers xylazine test strips for wholesale orders. CDC+4DanceSafe+4Bunk Police+4
- **Bunk Police**
    - Offers a wide range of reagent kits (e.g., Marquis, Mandelin) and Fentanyl test strips for various substances—from MDMA and LSD to novel research chemicals. DanceSafe+8Bunk Police+8TIME+8
- **BTNX Rapid Response™ Fentanyl Test Strips**
    - A highly accurate, quick dipstick test (as fast as 1 minute) for fentanyl detection; praised for its sensitivity in independent studies. btnx.com
- **State & Public Health Programs**
    - Some state harm-reduction programs (e.g., New York's Office of Addiction Services and Supports) distribute **free drug test**

strips (such as fentanyl- and xylazine-strips) through mobile outreach. Herald Sun+4Network for Public Health Law+4CDC+4AP News+3Addiction Services and Supports+3Network for Public Health Law+3

- Fentanyl and xylazine test strips have also been legally declassified as paraphernalia in certain states, like Mississippi, allowing broader access. AP News

Commercial & Retail Products

Portable strip test for fentanyl in powders/pills/liquids
Ütest Fentanyl Substance Strip Kit
$13.00
Ütest Drug Testing

Comprehensive 16-panel urine screening including fentanyl
Prime Screen 16-Panel Multi-Drug Test Kit
$203.99
Prime Screen

Highlights:

- **Ütest Fentanyl Substance Strip Kit**
  Designed to detect fentanyl in solid or liquid substances (powders, pills, liquids). Includes all necessary items—pipette, gloves, instructions. Useful for quick, on-the-spot drug screening.
- **Prime Screen 16-Panel Multi-Drug Test Kit**
  A broad-spectrum urine test kit that screens for 16 different substances—including amphetamines, cocaine, MDMA, opioids, and fentanyl itself. Great for comprehensive testing.

Additional Options (Commercial Drug Tests)

Other readily available options include:

- **Walgreens At-Home Drug Test Kits**
  Available in 4-, 7-, and 14-panel formats, plus specific tests for THC or cocaine detection. AmazonWalgreens
- **Touch&Know Multi-Drug Test Kit**
  Online seller (e.g., Amazon) offering a 30-substance general screening kit—though customer reviews note mixed accuracy. Amazon
- **10-Panel Dip Drug Testing Kit**
  An FDA-cleared, SAMHSA-approved instant urine screening device for 10 common drugs/metabolites. BioMed Central+15Amazon+15Amazon+15

Summary & Recommendations

Provider Type	Strengths	Considerations
Nonprofit Kits	Community-driven, harm-reduction-focused	May require ordering directly from nonprofit shops
Commercial Kits	Easily purchased, useful for self-screening	Some focus on urine (not substance purity); vary in accuracy
Public Health Programs	Often **free** and accessible locally	Availability varies by location, often limited to fentanyl/xylazine strips

- If your goal is to **identify potential contaminants or confirm substance identity**, reagent kits (DanceSafe, Bunk Police) or fentanyl/xylazine strips are more appropriate.
- For **screening multiple drugs via urine tests** (e.g., for employment or personal health checks), commercial panel kits from Walgreens, Prime Screen, or Ütest fit the bill.

In Summary

- **Best harm-reduction tools:** DanceSafe and Bunk Police reagent strips, plus BTNX Fentanyl strips.
- **Convenient consumer options:** Walgreens or Amazon multi-panel screens, or direct kits from Ütest and Prime Screen.
- **Access via public health:** Check your local harm-reduction or health departments for free fentanyl/xylazine strip distribution.

Bottom line:

Let me close with this- I remain absolutely convinced: crystal meth has been, directly or indirectly, responsible for more deaths in the gay community than AIDS ever was—and yet unlike HIV 30 years into this epidemic we haven't made any progress. Overdose deaths involving psychostimulants like methamphetamine climbed from roughly 23,800 in 2020 to over 32,500 in 2021—an alarming upward trajectory in a crisis that remains largely ignored and those are just the deaths that are directly attributable. Not the suicides, or the heart attacks, or the bizarre acts from paranoia or the AIDS deaths and even murders that were 100% related to meth use. While HIV has received decades of attention, research funding, has effective treatments, and advocacy; meth addiction—still has no effective pharmacologic treatment after thirty years—even as it devastates lives, sexual health, and community cohesion. Tom of P-Town is judgment-free, but make no mistake: this drug is the single most dangerous thing a gay man can encounter. The scale of its harm—both in terms of physical health and social ruin—is staggering, and we owe it to our community to finally treat it with the urgency it demands and if you aren't already engaged with it-please give it a hard pass.

Additionally, GHB has razor-thin safety margins so be careful if you are going to use it. Testing your substances, pacing doses, protecting your sexual health, and knowing where to get support are essential harm-reduction steps. Again, at Tom of P-Town my recommendation to every patient is to never do crystal meth not once, not ever.

Addiction & Support Resources

A quick way to self-screen for possible addiction is to ask yourself three simple questions: **(1)** Have I tried to cut back and found I couldn't? **(2)** Am I spending more time, money, or energy on drugs or alcohol than I want to? **(3)** Have my relationships, work, or health suffered because of my use? If you answer "yes" to even one of these, it may be a sign that substances are taking more control than you'd like. That doesn't mean you've failed—it means it might be time to get support. Free and confidential resources include the **SAMHSA National Helpline (1-800-662-HELP)**, local LGBTQ-affirming health clinics, and peer groups like **Crystal Meth Anonymous (CMA)**, **SMART Recovery**, or your local recovery community centers. Reaching out is not weakness—it's the first strong step toward getting your life back in balance.

- **SAMHSA Helpline (US):** 1-800-662-HELP (24/7, free, confidential)

- **Trevor Project (LGBTQ+ youth):** 1-866-488-7386 or text START to 678-678
- **Crystal Meth Anonymous (crystalmeth.org):** Peer meetings, online/in-person
- **SMART Recovery (smartrecovery.org):** Evidence-based addiction recovery
- **Local LGBTQ+ clinics:** Often offer PrEP, DoxyPEP, STI testing, and substance use counseling

Chemsex Overdose & Emergency Response Guide

If in doubt: Call 911 (or local emergency number). Don't wait — minutes matter.
Place the person on their side in the **recovery position** if unconscious but breathing.

🚨 GHB / GBL

Warning signs:

- Unconsciousness
- Slow or irregular breathing
- Vomiting while unconscious
- Seizures

What to do:

- Place in **recovery position** (on their side, head tilted back)
- Keep airway clear — don't leave them on their back
- Call emergency services immediately

- **Do NOT "let them sleep it off"** — death can occur silently

💉 Methamphetamine ("Tina"), Mephedrone, Cocaine

Warning signs:

- Chest pain, racing or irregular heartbeat
- Severe anxiety, paranoia, hallucinations
- Seizures
- Overheating (hot, dry skin, confusion)

What to do:

- Move to a **cool, quiet place**
- Loosen clothing, cool with damp cloths or ice packs (armpits, groin, neck)
- Sip water or electrolytes if awake & alert
- Call emergency services if chest pain, seizure, or collapse

❄□ Ketamine

Warning signs:

- Loss of control or coordination
- Unconsciousness
- Slow/shallow breathing
- Hallucinations, agitation, or confusion

What to do:

- Keep in safe area — prevent falls or injury

- If unconscious: recovery position
- Monitor breathing closely
- Call emergency services if they don't wake or breathing slows

⚠️ Opioid Adulteration (Fentanyl in meth, cocaine, ketamine)

Warning signs:

- Slow or stopped breathing
- Blue lips/fingernails
- Pinpoint pupils
- Unresponsive

What to do:

- Call 911 immediately
- Administer **naloxone (Narcan)** if available
- Rescue breaths if not breathing (1 every 5 seconds)
- Keep monitoring until EMS arrives — repeat naloxone in 2–3 min if needed

□ General Safety Tips

- **Don't use alone** — have a buddy system
- **Track doses & times** (esp. with GHB/GBL)
- **Carry naloxone (Narcan)** — available at most pharmacies & harm reduction centers
- Know your local **Good Samaritan laws** — in many places, calling 911 for an overdose protects you from prosecution for personal use

✅ **Quick Kit to Bring to Chemsex Events:**

- Condoms, lube, gloves
- Fentanyl test strips, reagent kits
- Naloxone (Narcan)
- Oral syringes for GHB dosing
- Sterile needles if injecting
- Water/electrolytes, snacks
- First aid basics (gloves, gauze, antiseptic wipes)

Chapter 15. Alcohol, Cannabis & Prescription Meds – Mixing Risks and Moderation Plans (MSM Focus)

When it comes to alcohol, cannabis, and prescription medications, most people already know the risks—overuse, mixing substances, and self-medicating can all backfire. But two substances deserve closer attention in our community: cannabis and benzodiazepines.

Cannabis is now a **multi-billion dollar industry**—the U.S. legal market alone is projected to reach nearly **$45 billion in 2025**. Benzodiazepines, meanwhile, remain among the most commonly prescribed classes of psychiatric medication, with more than **92 million prescriptions written annually in the U.S.** Together, these drugs represent big business, and that financial weight matters when it comes to the kind of research that gets published.

Both cannabis and benzos are widely used by men who have sex with men to cope with anxiety. And to be fair, they can provide **short-term relief**: a joint might take the edge off; a Xanax can stop a panic attack. But here's the catch: **neither works as a long-term anxiety solution.** Cannabis can worsen anxiety and depression with heavy use or withdrawal. Benzos carry well-documented risks of dependence, tolerance, and cognitive decline with long-term use.

And here's what's missing: despite their popularity, **high-quality, randomized controlled studies** on long-term anxiety management with cannabis or benzodiazepines simply aren't available—at least not studies free from **industry sponsorship** or commercial interest. Much of the evidence we do have comes from companies and organizations that profit from keeping patients tied to these substances. The result is that clinicians and patients alike are left without clear, unbiased data to guide safe, long-term care.

So, while both cannabis and benzos can feel helpful in the moment, neither belongs in the category of *true anxiety medications.* They are temporary patches that can set up a cycle of dependence and worsening symptoms once the short-term effect wears off.

This chapter isn't here to shame use, but to help you see these substances for what they are—multi-billion-dollar industries selling short-term fixes without long-term answers. What follows is a realistic look at safer strategies, moderation plans, and evidence-based treatments that actually support mental health in the long run.

Cannabis and benzos may soothe anxiety now, but both can exacerbate it in the long run—especially during withdrawal. That's alarming, because neither has solid evidence supporting long-term anxiety management. So while they're commonly used, they're not actually anxiety treatments—they're temporary patches.

Evidence Snapshot

Cannabis & Anxiety Risks:

- Longitudinal data show cannabis use is associated with **a 25–28% higher odds** of developing anxiety disorders over time (OR ≈ 1.25; 95% CI: 1.01–1.54)

- **Daily or near-daily cannabis use** increases the risk of developing anxiety or depressive disorders, disrupts dopamine-driven pleasure responses, and may impair emotional regulation
- Cannabis dependence affects **approximately 9–20%** of users—particularly daily users—with associated withdrawal symptoms like irritability, anxiety, insomnia, and depression
- Self-medicating cannabis users, especially those consuming high-THC doses, are at **higher risk of paranoia and psychotic symptoms** compared to recreational users

Benzodiazepines & Long-Term Harms:

- Though benzos are effective short-term, **long-term use beyond 2–4 weeks** is linked to cognitive impairment, worsened sleep architecture, dependency, and worsening psychiatric symptoms over time
- Users are at increased risk for addiction, withdrawal symptoms, **cognitive decline**, vehicle accidents, and **hip fractures** (especially in older adults)—driving while on benzos carries risk similar to alcohol intoxication
- Up to **15–44%** of long-term users develop physical dependence; withdrawal symptoms can be severe—anxiety, panic, perceptual disturbances, and even seizures or suicidal behaviors.
- Neurotoxic effects have been documented: synapse loss and lasting cognitive impairments—shown in animal models and supported by patient experiences

Putting It All Together

- **Cannabis and benzos may soothe in the moment,** but they often **create or worsen anxiety over time,** especially when use becomes regular or stops abruptly.
- Neither substance is supported by strong evidence for **safe, effective long-term anxiety treatment.**
- That makes them *not* actual anxiety medications—just relief that can turn into risk.

This isn't about judgment—it's a reality check. If you're using cannabis or benzos to self-manage anxiety, take a breath—and keep reading. The rest of this chapter explores how to approach these substances with awareness, create moderation plans, and discover healthier, sustainable ways to manage anxiety—together.

Why This Matters in MSM Health

Alcohol, cannabis, and prescription medications are common in many people's lives. But in MSM communities, these substances can play an even bigger role in social spaces—bars, clubs, sex parties, Pride events, or intimate encounters. Sometimes they help with relaxation, confidence, or connection. Sometimes they're used to manage stigma, anxiety, or trauma.

Understanding how alcohol, cannabis, and prescription meds interact can help you enjoy yourself while reducing risks to your health, safety, and relationships.

Alcohol

Common Contexts for MSM

- **Bars and clubs** are often central social spaces in gay culture. Alcohol is almost always present.
- **Sexual encounters** may involve drinking to reduce anxiety or inhibition.
- **Pride and circuit parties** often normalize heavy drinking.

Risks

- Alcohol lowers inhibitions, which can increase risky sexual behavior (condomless sex, multiple partners, forgetting PrEP/PEP).
- Chronic heavy use can worsen depression and anxiety—both already higher in MSM due to minority stress.
- Alcohol dependence is more common among MSM compared to heterosexual men.

Dangerous Interactions

- **With ED meds (Viagra, Cialis):** alcohol can worsen dizziness, fainting, and unsafe blood pressure drops.
- **With HIV meds:** heavy drinking stresses the liver, which already works hard metabolizing ART.
- **With SSRIs or other psych meds:** alcohol blunts the benefits of treatment and can worsen mood swings.
- **With benzodiazepines or opioids:** overdose risk is very high.

Safer Use

- Hydrate between drinks and eat beforehand.

- Know your "triggers": if alcohol tends to lead you into risky sex or missed meds, plan alternatives.
- Have an exit plan from parties or bars before you get too intoxicated.

Cannabis

Common Contexts for MSM

- Used to reduce anxiety before sex or social events.
- Can heighten sensuality, increase touch sensitivity, and lower inhibitions.
- Edibles are popular at parties; smoking/vaping is common in group or one-on-one encounters.

Risks

- **Anxiety paradox:** While many people reach for cannabis to calm nerves, studies show it can just as often **trigger or worsen anxiety and panic**, especially in higher-THC strains.
- **Dependence:** Regular use can create psychological dependence, with irritability, insomnia, or restlessness when stopping.
- **Cognition:** Chronic use may impair memory, focus, and motivation.
- **Lungs:** Smoking adds lung irritation, which can compound HIV, asthma, or other chronic conditions.

📌 Cannabis Myths vs. Facts

Proven in studies (evidence supports):

- Chronic pain relief (especially nerve-related pain).
- Chemotherapy-related nausea and vomiting.
- Appetite stimulation in HIV and cancer-related weight loss.
- Seizure control (CBD in certain rare seizure disorders).

Less proven / mixed evidence:

- Anxiety: sometimes short-term relief, but often worsens or triggers anxiety.
- Sleep: may help with falling asleep, but disrupts sleep quality long-term.
- Depression: no strong evidence; heavy use linked to worse symptoms.
- Glaucoma: lowers eye pressure only briefly—not a practical treatment.

Myths:

- "Cannabis is harmless." (It carries real dependence and mental health risks.)
- "Cannabis cures cancer." (No reliable clinical evidence supports this.)
- "CBD fixes everything." (Only proven for certain seizures; other claims are unproven.)

Better Treatments in Some Cases

If you're using cannabis mainly for:

- **Anxiety:** Consider SSRIs, SNRIs, or cognitive behavioral therapy (CBT). Non-addictive meds like buspirone may help.

- **Sleep:** Safer long-term options include melatonin, better sleep hygiene, or short-term use of approved sleep aids.
- **Depression:** Antidepressants, exercise, and therapy have much stronger evidence.
- **Sexual anxiety:** Mindfulness, therapy, or adjusting ED medications may be safer and more effective than cannabis.

Dangerous Interactions

- **With ED meds:** cannabis can increase heart rate and blood pressure changes, adding strain.
- **With HIV meds:** generally low interaction risk, but some antiretrovirals are metabolized by the same liver enzymes as THC/CBD—levels may shift unpredictably.
- **With sedatives:** drowsiness, confusion, falls.

Safer Use

- Choose lower-THC, higher-CBD products if you want less anxiety and paranoia.
- Start low, go slow with edibles—overdosing is common and miserable.
- Choose non-smoking routes (edibles, tinctures, vaping) to avoid lung harm.
- If mixing cannabis and alcohol, remember that alcohol intensifies THC's effects.
- Never drive or operate machinery while high—also avoid risky anal play while too intoxicated to feel pain or damage.

Benzodiazepines (Xanax, Ativan, Klonopin, Valium)

What They're For

Benzodiazepines ("benzos") are sedative medications that can be very effective for **short-term** use: treating acute panic attacks, severe anxiety episodes, seizures, or short-term insomnia.

Problems With Long-Term Use in MSM

- **Dependence & Addiction:** Benzos are highly addictive; tolerance builds quickly, leading to higher doses for the same effect.
- **Mental Health:** While they calm anxiety short term, long-term use often **worsens depression and anxiety**, creating a cycle of dependence.
- **Sexual Health:** Sedation and memory blackouts can increase the risk of unsafe or non-consensual sex. Some men report combining benzos with sex to "numb out" from trauma, which creates further emotional distance.
- **Community impact:** Studies show higher-than-average benzodiazepine misuse among MSM, often combined with alcohol or party drugs.

Age Risks

- **Older adults (over 55–60):** Benzos increase risk of falls, fractures, confusion, and memory problems. Guidelines strongly discourage long-term use in this age group.

Why SSRIs Are Better Long-Term

- SSRIs and SNRIs (like sertraline, escitalopram, or venlafaxine) treat the underlying brain chemistry of anxiety and depression.
- They don't cause tolerance or dependence.
- They improve both mood and anxiety symptoms over time, while benzos only suppress symptoms temporarily.

Coming Off Benzodiazepines

- **Never stop suddenly.** Stopping abruptly can trigger life-threatening seizures, severe anxiety, or hallucinations.
- **Tapering is essential.** Doctors usually recommend a slow wean over weeks to months, sometimes switching to a longer-acting benzo before tapering down.
- **Exploring alternatives:** SSRIs, therapy, non-addictive meds (buspirone, hydroxyzine), and mindfulness practices can replace chronic benzo use.

☞ If you're currently on chronic benzodiazepine treatment: talk to your provider about a **gradual taper plan** and ask what other treatments might serve your needs better long-term.

Prescription Medications in MSM Health

HIV Medications (ART/PrEP/PEP)

- Heavy drinking can harm the liver and increase missed doses.

- Cannabis has few direct interactions but may worsen adherence if overused.

ED Medications (Viagra, Cialis, Levitra)

- Alcohol + ED meds = higher risk of fainting or unsafe blood pressure drops.
- Cannabis can worsen dizziness when combined with ED meds.

Performance-Enhancing Medications

- **Testosterone or anabolic steroids:** alcohol worsens liver strain; cannabis may worsen mood swings.
- **Finasteride (for hair loss):** alcohol and cannabis don't directly interact in formal drug to drug interactions with this, but mood effects can overlap.

Mixing in MSM Social & Sexual Settings

- **Crossfading (alcohol + cannabis):** common at parties, but increases nausea, dizziness, and blackouts.
- **Alcohol + ED meds:** risky because both affect blood pressure.
- **Sedatives (like benzos) + alcohol/cannabis:** can cause blackout sex, inability to consent, or overdose.
- **"Party & Play" contexts:** alcohol and cannabis may be mixed with stimulants (meth, cocaine, mephedrone). This greatly increases risk of overdose and risky sex.

Moderation & Safer Use Plans for MSM

✓☐ **Know your setting**—if you're drinking at a sex party, consider whether it might lead to unsafe sex choices.

✓☐ **Use reminders**—set phone alarms for PrEP/PEP/HIV meds before events with drinking.

✓☐ **Buddy system**—go out with a trusted friend who can help if you're too intoxicated.

✓☐ **Know your meds**—especially if you're on HIV treatment, ED meds, or psych meds.

✓☐ **Alternate nights**—don't always tie sex to drinking or cannabis; try sober intimacy too.

When to Seek Help

- Drinking/smoking before *every* sexual encounter.
- Memory gaps around sex ("I don't remember what happened").
- Missing HIV meds, PrEP, or other prescriptions because of use.
- Feeling unable to cut back even when it's hurting relationships, health, or work.
- Depending on benzos daily and feeling unable to stop.

Online Screening Tools

- **AUDIT (Alcohol Use Disorders Identification Test):**

  ☞ https://www.niaaa.nih.gov/alcohols-effects-health/interactive-alcohol-screener

- **ASSIST (Alcohol, Smoking and Substance Involvement Screening Test):**
  ☞ https://www.who.int/tools/assist-instrument
- **CAGE Questionnaire (Alcohol):**
  ☞ https://alcoholscreen.org
- **Drug Abuse Screening Test (DAST-10):**
  ☞ https://cde.drugabuse.gov/instrument/f1d3f4a1-4044-74f8-e040-bb89ad433d69

Why Screening Matters for MSM

- **Sexual safety:** Substance use may increase the risk of condomless sex, missed PrEP doses, or forgetting to use PEP.
- **Mental health:** MSM are at higher risk for anxiety, depression, and trauma—all of which can be masked by alcohol, cannabis, or benzos.
- **Non-judgmental step:** Screening can be a first private step before deciding if you'd like professional support.

Resources for MSM

- **SAMHSA National Helpline:** 1-800-662-HELP — https://www.samhsa.gov/find-help/national-helpline
- **The Trevor Project (LGBTQ youth crisis support):** https://www.thetrevorproject.org
- **Gay & Sober (peer support and community events):** https://gayandsober.org
- **DanceSafe (harm reduction & drug checking):** https://dancesafe.org

- Local LGBTQ+ community health centers and HIV clinics often provide **confidential screening, counseling, and support programs**.

⚠️ High-Risk Combos at a Glance

Combination	Risks
Alcohol + Benzodiazepines	Blackouts, respiratory depression, overdose, death
Alcohol + Opioids	Very high overdose risk, slowed breathing, fatal events
Alcohol + ED Meds	Dangerous drops in blood pressure, fainting, unsafe sex scenarios
Alcohol + Cannabis	Stronger impairment, vomiting, blackouts ("crossfade")
Cannabis + Sedatives	Extreme drowsiness, falls, confusion
Benzodiazepines + Stimulants (e.g., meth, cocaine)	Dangerous heart stress, seizures, overdose risk
Benzodiazepines + Chronic Use	Dependence, withdrawal seizures, worsening depression/anxiety
Cannabis + Heavy Alcohol	Poor judgment, unsafe sex, medication non-adherence

✨ **Bottom line for MSM:** Alcohol, cannabis, and benzodiazepines may feel like tools for easing stress, fitting in socially, or enhancing sex — but the risks, especially with mixing, are real. Knowing the science, recognizing the myths, and exploring healthier alternatives (like SSRIs for anxiety) puts you in control of both your health and your pleasure.

Chapter 16. Recognizing Trouble – Overdose Signs, Serotonin Syndrome, and When to Call 911

Why This Matters in MSM Health

One of my past patients, a man with a history of occasional methamphetamine use, was prescribed quetiapine (Seroquel) by a well-meaning nurse practitioner to help with sleep and mood. On its own, quetiapine does not cause serotonin syndrome. But in combination with other serotonergic agents—like methamphetamine—it can tip the balance toward dangerous neurochemical overload. After a weekend of partying, he developed agitation, tremor, confusion, and rapid fluctuations in blood pressure and heart rate. He went to the emergency department, but the possibility of serotonin syndrome was never considered. Instead, his symptoms were attributed to "just being high," and he was discharged once the acute agitation began to wane.

This case illustrates why serotonin syndrome can be easily overlooked in the ER, particularly when providers are not aware of a patient's recreational drug use. Serotonin syndrome is a potentially life-threatening condition caused by excess serotonin in the central nervous system. While it's classically linked to prescription medications such as SSRIs, SNRIs, MAO inhibitors, certain opioids (like tramadol, fentanyl, or meperidine), and even over-the-counter products like dextromethorphan, it can also occur when those agents are combined with stimulants or recreational drugs. Because the presentation can mimic intoxication, withdrawal, or other psychiatric and medical emergencies, the diagnosis is often missed unless clinicians think to ask the right questions.

That's why this chapter exists. Knowing the warning signs of overdose of drugs, understanding what serotonin syndrome and other overdose symptoms look like, and recognizing when to call 911 can literally save lives. For men who use party drugs—or who may be prescribed medications that interact with them—awareness is the most powerful safety net. Most importantly, err on the side of caution- if something doesn't feel right call 911 and get an ambulance.

Substance use can sometimes cross a line from fun or manageable into a medical emergency. Overdose doesn't only happen with heroin or fentanyl — alcohol, GHB, benzos, MDMA, cocaine, meth, and even prescription antidepressants can all cause life-threatening reactions.

In MSM communities, overdoses often happen at sex parties, clubs, or when mixing drugs to manage sexual anxiety. Recognizing warning signs early can save your life or someone else's.

Recognizing General Overdose Signs CALL 911!!

Alcohol & Sedatives (including GHB, sleeping pills)

- Extreme drowsiness or inability to stay awake
- Slow or irregular breathing
- Limp body, unable to be woken
- Pale, clammy, or bluish skin
- Vomiting while unconscious

Key Danger: Respiratory depression (breathing slows or stops).

Benzodiazepines (Xanax, Ativan, Klonopin, Valium)

- Extreme sleepiness, difficult to arouse
- Slurred speech, poor coordination, staggering
- Confusion or memory blackouts
- Shallow or slowed breathing (especially if mixed with alcohol or opioids)
- Very low blood pressure, weak pulse
- Loss of consciousness or coma

Key Danger: Alone, benzo overdoses are rarely fatal — but combined with alcohol, opioids, or other sedatives, they can easily stop breathing and be deadly.

📌 **Call-Out: Benzodiazepine Dependence vs. Overdose**

Dependence (long-term creeping problem):

- Daily or frequent benzo use
- Needing higher doses for the same effect
- Using to sleep every night
- Feeling anxious, shaky, or unable to function without them
- Memory problems or missing big chunks of time

Overdose (acute emergency):

- Cannot stay awake or respond
- Very slow or shallow breathing
- Slurred speech, unable to walk straight
- Loss of consciousness
- Danger highest when mixed with alcohol or opioids

☞ If it looks like overdose → call 911 immediately.
☞ If it looks like dependence → talk with a provider about tapering safely.

Opioids (oxycodone, heroin, fentanyl)

- Very slow or no breathing
- Pinpoint pupils
- Blue lips or fingertips
- Snoring or gurgling sounds ("death rattle")
- Unresponsive to voice or pain

Key Danger: Fatal respiratory arrest — requires naloxone immediately.

Stimulants (meth, cocaine, mephedrone)

- Extreme agitation or paranoia
- Seizures or convulsions
- Very high heart rate or chest pain
- Overheating, profuse sweating, or collapse
- Sudden confusion, hallucinations

Key Danger: Heart attack, stroke, or sudden collapse.

MDMA (Ecstasy/Molly)

- High body temperature, overheating
- Sweating, shaking, muscle cramps
- Confusion or paranoia

- Seizures, collapse, loss of consciousness

Key Danger: Heat stroke, dehydration, serotonin syndrome.

Serotonin Syndrome

What it is: A potentially fatal reaction when serotonin levels get too high in the brain.

Can be triggered by:

- **SSRIs/SNRIs (sertraline, venlafaxine, escitalopram, etc.)**
- **MAOIs (rare but high risk)**
- **Tricyclic antidepressants (TCAs)**
- **Other psychiatric meds** that raise serotonin (like trazodone, mirtazapine, lithium)
- **MDMA, meth, mephedrone** (alone or mixed with above meds)
- **Certain opioids** (tramadol, fentanyl, meperidine)
- **Over-the-counter meds** like dextromethorphan (cough syrup) and supplements like St. John's Wort

Signs:

- Agitation, restlessness, confusion
- Rapid heart rate, high blood pressure
- Muscle twitching, tremors, clonus (jerky movements)
- Sweating, shivering, fever
- Severe: seizures, irregular heartbeat, loss of consciousness

When to act: Call 911 if you see these signs — serotonin syndrome can progress fast.

📝 Self-Checklist: Could This Be Serotonin Syndrome?

If you've recently taken prescription antidepressants, meth, MDMA, or other drugs that affect serotonin, use this quick guide. If you check **more than one** of these boxes, call 911 or go to the ER right away.

Body Signs

- ☐ My muscles are stiff, jerking, or twitching uncontrollably.
- ☐ I'm shaking, sweating heavily, or running a high fever.
- ☐ My pupils are very large and my eyes keep darting around.
- ☐ My heart is racing or my blood pressure feels very high or very low.

Mental/Behavioral Signs

- ☐ I feel extremely agitated, restless, or anxious in a way that feels out of control.
- ☐ I'm confused, disoriented, or having trouble thinking clearly.
- ☐ I see or hear things that aren't there.

GI & Other Clues

- ☐ I have bad nausea, vomiting, or diarrhea that came on suddenly.
- ☐ My body feels overheated and I can't cool down.

⚠️ **Emergency Rule of Thumb**:
If symptoms appear **suddenly**, are **getting worse**, or involve **confusion, fever, or severe muscle stiffness**, **call 911 immediately**.

When to Call 911

Call 911 right away if:

- Someone is unconscious and won't wake up
- Breathing is slow, irregular, or stopped
- **Any seizure happens** — whether it stops on its own or not
- Chest pain, collapse, or sudden severe confusion
- Signs of serotonin syndrome (confusion, tremors, fever, seizures)
- Lips, skin, or nails turn blue

Warning Signs of Growing Dependence

Alcohol

- Drinking before or during most sexual encounters
- Blackouts, memory gaps
- Needing more alcohol for the same effect
- Drinking despite worsened depression or relationships

Cannabis

- Using daily for relaxation or socializing
- Feeling anxious or irritable without it
- Trouble sleeping or eating when stopping
- Relying on it for every sexual encounter

Benzodiazepines

- Needing higher doses to feel calm
- Using benzos for sleep every night
- Memory problems, sedation interfering with life
- Feeling unable to stop despite wanting to
- Using with alcohol or stimulants to balance effects

Stimulants (meth, cocaine, mephedrone)

- Binging for longer than planned
- Sexual encounters only happening when using
- Cravings and "crash depression" after use
- Missing work, meds, or commitments
- Increased risky sex behaviors

Drug Testing as Harm Reduction

- **Fentanyl test strips:** Detect contamination in cocaine, pills, meth, MDMA.
- **Reagent kits (DanceSafe, Energy Control):** Identify MDMA, adulterants, stimulants.
- **Mail-in lab services:** Some organizations allow small anonymous samples for full analysis.

Testing doesn't guarantee safety but reduces risk of unexpected adulterants.

Recovery Options

12-Step (AA, NA, CMA)

- Peer-based, structured, spiritual emphasis.
- Widely available, including LGBTQ-friendly meetings.

SMART Recovery

- Secular, based on science and CBT tools.
- Focuses on empowerment and coping skills.

Buddhist/Mindfulness-Based Recovery (Refuge Recovery, Recovery Dharma)

- Meditation, compassion, and community.
- Non-theistic and welcoming to LGBTQ+ communities.

Therapy-Based Approaches

- **CBT:** manage triggers, reframe thoughts.
- **Trauma therapy:** especially relevant in MSM where trauma often drives use.
- **Medication-assisted treatment:** buprenorphine, naltrexone, methadone for opioids; SSRIs instead of chronic benzos.

LGBTQ+ Specific Recovery Groups

- Local LGBTQ centers, "Gay & Sober," and online support networks provide affirming spaces.

Good Samaritan Laws

Most states (including Massachusetts) protect you from arrest for simple possession if you call 911 during an overdose.

Bottom Line for MSM

Overdoses happen — and dependence can creep in slowly, even when you don't expect it. Recognizing early signs, testing what you use, and knowing recovery options give you choices and control.

If you ever wonder, *"Is this getting out of hand?"* — that's the first signal to check in with yourself or talk to a trusted provider.

⚠︎□ Emergency Checklist (Cut-out Box)

Call 911 if:

- Unconscious, not waking up
- Slow, irregular, or stopped breathing
- **Any seizure**
- Blue lips or skin
- Overheating, confusion, tremors (possible serotonin syndrome)
- Chest pain, sudden collapse

While waiting:

- Give address first
- Say: "They're unresponsive and not breathing normally."
- Recovery position if unconscious but breathing
- Naloxone if opioids suspected
- Cool if overheating

Warning Signs of Dependence

Alcohol

- Needing more to feel the same effect
- Blackouts or missing time
- Drinking before/after every sexual encounter

Cannabis

- Using daily for relaxation
- Irritable or anxious without it
- Relying on it for sex or sleep

Benzodiazepines

- Needing higher doses to stay calm
- Daily reliance for sleep
- Memory gaps, sedation affecting life

Stimulants

- Using longer or more often than planned
- Sex only enjoyable with stimulants
- Craving/crash cycles disrupting life

☞ If you see yourself in these patterns, consider talking to a trusted provider, using online screening tools, or exploring recovery options.

Chapter 17. Body Image Pressures, Muscle Dysmorphia & Anorexia

Why This Matters in MSM Health

If you asked me what the single most common lab test my patients request, I wouldn't hesitate: it's testosterone. Week after week, men in their late 20s or early 30s—healthy, muscular, with no real signs or symptoms of hypogonadism—ask me to check their "T levels." Often, the unspoken hope is that the numbers will come back low enough to justify supplementation, giving them a doctor-approved shortcut to faster muscle growth.

This isn't surprising. In the gay community especially, there's enormous social pressure to maintain a lean, muscular body. Research shows that gay and bisexual men report higher rates of body dissatisfaction than their heterosexual peers, and they are more likely to engage in extreme dieting, excessive exercise, or the misuse of performance-enhancing drugs. In one large U.S. survey, up to **42% of gay men** reported being dissatisfied with their bodies, compared with about 17% of heterosexual men. Other studies suggest that as many as **one in five gay men** may experience disordered eating behaviors at some point, with muscle dysmorphia—sometimes called "bigorexia"—becoming increasingly common.

The consequences extend beyond physical health. When men feel they don't measure up to the sculpted physiques celebrated in gay media and dating apps, the result can be shame, low self-esteem, and even depression. Patients come to me convinced that low testosterone is the culprit, when in reality, what they are feeling is the heavy weight of comparison. And because the idea of "fixing" body image with hormones or supplements can be so alluring, it creates a dangerous cycle that sometimes ends in unnecessary medication use, risky anabolic steroid practices, or worsening mental health.

This chapter will explore how body image pressures uniquely affect men who have sex with men, unpack the rise of muscle dysmorphia and eating disorders in this community, and provide tools for recognizing unhealthy patterns before they spiral into something more dangerous

Many men in MSM communities feel intense pressure to look a certain way — muscular, lean, youthful, and sexually appealing. Gym culture, social media, pornography, and dating apps can amplify these expectations. For some, working out and fitness are healthy and affirming. For others, body image pressures can become overwhelming, leading to risky behaviors like steroid misuse, compulsive exercise, restrictive eating, or even full-blown eating disorders.

Muscle dysmorphia and anorexia are two extremes on the same spectrum of body image distress — one focused on being "not big enough," the other on being "too big" and striving for extreme thinness. Both are serious mental health conditions that disproportionately affect MSM.

Body Image Pressures in MSM Communities

- **Gay & bi men are at higher risk** of body dissatisfaction compared to heterosexual men.
- **Media & porn** often idealize a narrow "type": lean, ripped, hairless, youthful.
- **Apps & social media** reinforce these ideals with shirtless profiles, gym selfies, and constant comparisons.

- **Age-related pressures:** Older MSM often feel invisible if they don't maintain a youthful body shape.
- **Intersectionality:** Men of color, trans men, and men with HIV may experience unique pressures (e.g., appearing "healthy" to counteract stigma).

Muscle Dysmorphia ("Bigorexia")

What it is: A form of body dysmorphic disorder (BDD) where someone feels small, weak, or "not muscular enough," even when they are objectively muscular.

Signs include:

- Feeling "too small" despite being muscular.
- Spending excessive time in the gym, missing social events or work.
- Strict, inflexible eating patterns (high protein obsession, fear of missing meals).
- Anxiety or depression if workouts are missed.
- Using anabolic steroids or risky supplements to try to achieve an "ideal."

Risks:

- Steroid use → heart disease, liver/kidney strain, infertility, mood swings.
- Overtraining → injuries, hormone imbalance.
- Mental health → anxiety, depression, isolation.

Anorexia Nervosa

What it is: An eating disorder marked by extreme restriction of food, fear of weight gain, and a distorted body image — feeling "too big" even when underweight.

Signs include:

- Severe food restriction or rigid dieting rules.
- Intense fear of gaining weight or being "soft."
- Obsession with calories, fasting, or "clean eating."
- Dramatic weight loss or dangerously low weight.
- Social withdrawal to avoid eating with others.
- Cold intolerance, fatigue, loss of libido.

Risks:

- Malnutrition → anemia, weakened immune system, hair loss, brittle bones.
- Heart complications → arrhythmias, heart failure.
- Hormonal issues → low testosterone, erectile dysfunction, infertility.
- High suicide risk.

Why MSM Are More Vulnerable

- **Cultural ideals:** Both hyper-muscularity and extreme leanness are prized in different gay subcultures.
- **Dating apps & porn:** Constant comparison intensifies body dissatisfaction.
- **Minority stress:** Trauma, stigma, and rejection can fuel disordered eating and body control behaviors.
- **HIV history:** In past decades, wasting was stigmatized — leading some men to equate being lean or muscular with "looking healthy."

📌 Sidebar: Healthy Body Diversity in MSM Communities

One powerful antidote to body image stress is remembering that MSM culture has a **rich diversity of body ideals** — not just one "perfect" type. Different subcultures celebrate different shapes and sizes:

- **Bears:** Larger, hairy men celebrated for strength, warmth, and masculinity.
- **Otters:** Lean but hairy men, fitting somewhere between twinks and bears.
- **Twinks:** Youthful, slim, often hairless men.
- **Daddies:** Older men, often prized for maturity, presence, and confidence.
- **Jocks, muscle men, gym bros:** Muscular men admired for fitness and power.
- **Chubs & chasers:** Communities that embrace larger bodies.

🌈 What this shows: desirability in MSM culture isn't monolithic — for every "type," there's a community that celebrates it.

Healthy Fitness vs. Disordered Body Image

- **Healthy fitness:** Exercise and nutrition support energy, confidence, and wellbeing.
- **Muscle dysmorphia:** Fitness becomes an obsession with endless muscle-building.
- **Anorexia:** Fitness and diet become tools for extreme restriction, shrinking, or control.

📝 Self-Check: Could I Have Body Dysmorphia?

If you often worry about your appearance, especially your muscles or body shape, this quick screen can help you reflect. Answer honestly:

Thoughts & Worries

- ☐ I spend a lot of time each day worrying that my body is too small, not muscular enough, or not lean enough.
- ☐ I compare my body to others constantly and usually feel worse afterward.
- ☐ I avoid social situations because I feel embarrassed about my appearance.

Behaviors

- ☐ I spend excessive time at the gym or exercising, even if I'm sick, injured, or exhausted.
- ☐ I stick to very strict diets or supplements because I'm afraid of losing muscle or gaining fat.
- ☐ I've thought about or used steroids, testosterone, or other substances to change how I look.

Feelings

- ☐ My mood (depression, anxiety, irritability) depends heavily on how I feel about my body.
- ☐ I feel distressed if I miss a workout or break my routine.
- ☐ My concerns about my body interfere with relationships, work, or daily life.

✅ **What to do:**

- If you checked **several boxes**, it may be a sign of **muscle dysmorphia or body dysmorphic disorder**.
- Remember: this checklist is **not a diagnosis**, but a signal that talking with a trusted provider or mental health professional could help.
- Support and treatment are available—whether that means therapy, support groups, or medical guidance.

Safer Approaches to Fitness & Body Image

Redefine Health

- Health is more than visible abs or being under a certain weight.

Train & Eat Smart

- Strength and cardio training support longevity and mood.
- A balanced diet with flexibility — not rigid rules — is healthiest.

Avoid Extremes

- Anabolic steroids and severe food restriction both carry high risks.

Mental Health Support

- Therapy (especially CBT) can help reframe distorted body thoughts.

Build Positive Culture

- Follow diverse, body-positive accounts on social media.
- Engage with friends and partners who value you beyond your appearance.

When to Seek Help

- Exercise, dieting, or body focus are interfering with relationships, work, or health.
- Feelings of shame, anxiety, or worthlessness dominate your body image.
- Use of steroids, clenbuterol, or diet pills.
- Weight loss or gain is causing physical health issues.
- Social isolation due to food or gym rituals.

Recovery & Support Options

- **Therapy:** CBT, eating disorder–focused therapy, or group therapy.
- **Eating disorder specialists:** Medical and nutritional support for safe recovery.
- **Support groups:** Some LGBTQ centers run groups on body image and disordered eating.
- **Medical care:** Monitoring hormones, heart, and nutrition.
- **Peer support:** Online and community body-positivity movements.

📋 Cut-Out Box: Warning Signs of Body Image Disorders

Muscle Dysmorphia

- Feeling too small even if muscular
- Gym prioritized over work/social life
- Obsessive high-protein diet
- Steroid/supplement misuse

Anorexia

- Severe food restriction
- Intense fear of gaining weight
- Very low weight, fatigue, loss of libido
- Social withdrawal to avoid meals

☞ Both are treatable. If you see yourself here, reach out for support.

Resources for Support

- **National Eating Disorders Association (NEDA)**
  Information, helpline, and screening tools for eating disorders.
  Website: https://www.nationaleatingdisorders.org
- **National Association for Males with Eating Disorders (NAMED)**
  Education and advocacy specific to men with eating disorders.
  Website: https://www.namedinc.org
- **Project HEAL**
  Offers support, mentorship, and treatment access for

people with eating disorders.
Website: https://www.theprojectheal.org

- **National Alliance for Eating Disorders**
Helpline and referral to treatment providers.
Website: https://www.allianceforeatingdisorders.com
- **The Trevor Project**
Crisis support for LGBTQ+ youth (not eating disorder–specific but relevant for younger MSM).
Website: https://www.thetrevorproject.org
- **Local LGBTQ+ Centers**
Many community centers offer body image or eating disorder support groups — search "[Your City] LGBTQ Center."

✨ **Bottom Line for MSM:** Body ideals in MSM culture can be intense — from the pressure to be ripped to the drive to stay thin. But chasing extremes can cost your health and happiness. Muscle dysmorphia and anorexia are real, serious conditions. Recovery is possible, and health looks different for every body.

Chapter 18. Gym Supplements & Steroids – What Works, What's Hype, What's Harmful

Walk into almost any gay gym or scroll through fitness influencers on social media, and one thing is impossible to miss: supplements are everywhere. Protein powders, pre-workouts, testosterone boosters, fat burners, creatine, herbal mixes—the list is endless. This isn't just a fitness fad; it's a multi-billion-dollar industry, one that thrives in no small part thanks to the buying power and cultural influence of the MSM community. For many men, supplements represent both hope and pressure: hope that the right pill or powder will get them closer to the body they want, and pressure to keep up with the sculpted ideals seen on apps, at clubs, and in media.

But here's the problem—unlike prescription medications, dietary supplements in the U.S. are **not tightly regulated**. They can be marketed with bold claims, often without rigorous safety or effectiveness studies. Worse, labels may not even match what's inside the bottle. Kratom, for example, has gained popularity in recent years as a "natural" performance enhancer and mood stabilizer, yet its unregulated use has been tied to seizures, liver injury, and even deaths. And the bodybuilding world still remembers the tragic 2017 death of a young man who ingested DNP (2,4-dinitrophenol), a so-called "fat-burning" chemical so toxic it's more commonly used as a pesticide than a supplement. Stories like this highlight how high the stakes can be when chasing performance or appearance goals with untested products.

This chapter doesn't exist to scare you away from every protein powder or vitamin. Some supplements—like creatine, whey protein, or vitamin D—have solid evidence supporting their safe and effective use when taken appropriately. But even the safest supplements can cause trouble when combined with prescription drugs, recreational substances, or preexisting medical conditions. Because these interactions are rarely studied, patients and even doctors may be blindsided by unexpected side effects.

That's why what follows is a balanced guide: which supplements actually work, which are mostly hype, and which can be outright harmful. Think of it as your roadmap through the crowded—and often confusing—world of gym supplements, with a reminder that **caution should always come first**.

Why This Matters in MSM Health

In MSM communities, gym culture often overlaps with dating culture, social circles, and even self-worth. A muscular, lean body is often seen as desirable, and many men pursue that ideal through **supplements, testosterone replacement therapy (TRT), anabolic steroids, or growth hormone**. But there's a big difference between **treating a real medical condition** like hypogonadism and **chasing fast gains with dangerous regimens**. This chapter helps you understand the difference.

Hypogonadism vs. "Wanting a Quick Fix"

True hypogonadism means your testes are not producing enough testosterone. This can be diagnosed with blood tests showing **low morning testosterone levels (usually**

measured between 7–10 AM) combined with symptoms such as:

- Fatigue, low energy
- Loss of muscle mass or strength
- Low libido or erectile dysfunction
- Depression, irritability
- Loss of body hair or small testes

In this case, TRT is medically appropriate.

What's not hypogonadism: Just wanting more muscles, faster recovery, or enhanced gym performance. Using TRT or anabolic steroids in this context is not treatment — it's enhancement, and carries major risks.

The Healthiest Form of TRT

If you do need TRT for true hypogonadism, the **safest and most physiologic replacement** is:

- **Topical testosterone gel applied in the morning.**
    - Mimics the natural **circadian rhythm** of testosterone (high in the morning, tapering at night).
    - Provides a steady, controlled dose.
    - Less risk of the extreme highs and lows seen with injections.

Why injections are problematic:

- Weekly or biweekly intramuscular injections create unnatural "peaks and valleys."
- Peaks → mood swings, acne, higher clotting risk.
- Valleys → fatigue, irritability, and libido loss.

- Injections are often pushed because they're profitable in clinics or easily abused in the black market.

☞ Bottom line: If you truly need TRT, ask your provider about morning topical gels as the first-line choice.

Steroid Cycling & Non-Physiologic Dosing

Many gym users take **anabolic steroid cycles** at doses far beyond medical replacement. These cycles may combine testosterone with other anabolic steroids (e.g., nandrolone, trenbolone).

Risks include:

- **Cardiovascular:** High blood pressure, high cholesterol, enlarged heart, heart attack, stroke.
- **Liver:** Toxicity, tumors, jaundice.
- **Kidneys:** Damage from chronic strain and high blood pressure.
- **Hormones:** Testicular shrinkage, infertility, breast tissue growth (gynecomastia).
- **Psychological:** Anger, paranoia, aggression ("roid rage"), depression after stopping.
- **Sexual:** Erectile dysfunction after withdrawal, dependence on exogenous testosterone.

Steroid cycling is **never safe** — it always carries long-term risks.

HGH (Human Growth Hormone) & Sermorelin

HGH (somatropin): Sometimes abused for muscle growth, fat loss, or "anti-aging."

Risks:

- Joint pain and swelling
- Carpal tunnel syndrome
- GI problems (bloating, abdominal growth)
- Increased risk of diabetes and cardiovascular disease
- Possible link to certain cancers (colorectal, prostate, lymphoma)

Sermorelin: A synthetic peptide that stimulates your body to release more growth hormone. Marketed as a "safer alternative," but:

- Very limited clinical data in adults
- Unknown long-term safety
- Similar risks as HGH due to overstimulation of IGF-1 pathways

☞ Bottom line: Neither HGH nor Sermorelin are safe or proven "youth" or muscle therapies.

Common Supplements: What Works vs. What's Hype

The supplement industry is a multi-billion dollar market — and much of it is hype. Here's a breakdown of what actually has evidence.

✓ Backed by Evidence (Safe & Effective for Most People)

- **Creatine monohydrate**: Improves strength, power, and muscle mass. Safest and most researched supplement.
- **Protein powders (whey, soy, pea)**: Help meet protein needs when diet falls short.
- **Caffeine**: Boosts performance, endurance, and alertness.
- **Beta-alanine**: May reduce fatigue in high-intensity exercise.

⚠️ Mixed Evidence or Limited Effect

- **BCAAs (branched-chain amino acids):** Overhyped; benefits are minimal if protein intake is already adequate.
- **Glutamine:** No strong evidence for muscle gain in healthy people.
- **Nitric oxide boosters (arginine, citrulline):** May improve blood flow and "pump," but effects are modest.

❌ Not Effective / Mostly Hype

- **Testosterone boosters (herbal blends like tribulus terrestris):** No real effect on testosterone.
- **Fat burners (green tea extract, raspberry ketones, "thermogenic" mixes):** Minimal benefit, often unsafe.
- **Pre-workouts with proprietary blends:** Often just caffeine plus fillers, with unknown safety.

🚫 Potentially Harmful

- **Prohormones / "designer steroids":** Sold as supplements, but really unregulated steroids.

- **SARMs (Selective Androgen Receptor Modulators):** Marketed as "safe steroids" but linked to liver toxicity, hormone disruption, and cardiovascular risk.

📌 **Call-Out Box: Myths vs. Facts**

Myth: "TRT injections are the gold standard for low testosterone."
Fact: Morning topical gels better mimic natural rhythms and are safer for long-term health.

Myth: "HGH is an anti-aging miracle."
Fact: HGH accelerates some aging processes and raises risks of diabetes, joint disease, and possibly cancer.

Myth: "Supplements are natural, so they're safe."
Fact: Many supplements are unregulated, under-tested, and can be contaminated with hidden steroids or stimulants.

Myth: "Anabolic steroids are safe if you cycle them carefully."
Fact: Even with cycles, long-term damage to the heart, liver, and brain is common and often permanent.

Harm Reduction if You Choose to Use Steroids

While we **do not recommend anabolic steroid use outside of medical TRT**, it's important to be realistic: some MSM will use black-market products. If you choose to do so, these strategies may help reduce (but not eliminate) the risks:

1. Source & Product Safety

- **Avoid underground labs and powders** — contamination is common.
- **Never share needles.** Use only sterile equipment. Sharing increases risk for HIV, hepatitis B, and hepatitis C.
- **Avoid veterinary products** (meant for animals) — often impure or dosed incorrectly.

2. Safer Use Practices

- **Lowest effective dose, shortest duration possible.**
- **Avoid stacking multiple anabolic compounds.**
- **Don't mix with alcohol, stimulants, or cocaine.**
- **Don't stop abruptly** if you've been on long-term steroids — withdrawal can cause severe depression, fatigue, and sexual dysfunction.

3. Medical Monitoring & Labs to Request

Ask your provider (ideally openly) for:

- **Every 3–6 months while on steroids:**
    - CBC
    - Lipid panel
    - Liver function tests (AST, ALT, bilirubin)
    - Kidney function (BUN, creatinine, eGFR)
    - Blood pressure and ECG
    - Hormone panel (testosterone, LH, FSH, estradiol, prolactin)
    - PSA (men over 40)
- **Once yearly:**
    - Echocardiogram (heart size/function)
    - Hepatitis B, C, and HIV testing (if injecting)

4. Harm Reduction for Coming Off Steroids

- **Do not stop cold turkey.**
- **Work with a provider** for tapering or medical restart protocols.
- **Expect mood changes, fatigue, and sexual dysfunction.** Plan for support during recovery.

📌 Call-Out Box: Harm Reduction Checklist

- Use sterile needles every time
- Don't share injection equipment
- Get labs every 3–6 months
- Monitor heart health with BP and ECG
- Be honest with your provider — many will help, not judge
- Plan for coming off: don't stop suddenly

Patient Vignette: Carlos' Story

Carlos, 34, started cycling testosterone and trenbolone at his gym buddy's suggestion. Within a few months he noticed rapid gains — bigger muscles, more confidence. But he also developed acne, mood swings, and insomnia. After stopping, his sex drive plummeted, he felt deeply depressed, and his doctor discovered his natural testosterone production had shut down.

With support, Carlos began harm reduction: he switched to sterile injection practices, started regular lab monitoring, and eventually worked with a provider to taper and restore natural hormone function. His story shows both the risks and the importance of having medical support — even if you're not ready to stop.

Psychological & Community Risks in MSM

- Steroid and supplement abuse is higher in MSM populations due to body image pressures.
- Risks include **depression, sexual dysfunction, and permanent infertility**.
- Black market drugs (including "underground labs") are common but often contaminated or mislabeled.
- Long-term use can lead to dependency: men feel they can't stop or they'll "lose their body" and social desirability.

Safer Fitness & Alternatives

- Work with a provider if you suspect hypogonadism; don't self-medicate.
- Stick with proven, safe supplements (creatine, protein, caffeine in moderation).
- Prioritize sleep, nutrition, and training consistency — the real drivers of progress.
- Seek therapy or peer support if you're struggling with body image pressures.

Resources

- **National Institute on Drug Abuse (NIDA):** https://nida.nih.gov/research-topics/anabolic-steroids
- **Mayo Clinic – Creatine:** https://www.mayoclinic.org/drugs-supplements-creatine/art-20347591

- **Endocrine Society – Testosterone Therapy Guidelines:** https://www.endocrine.org/clinical-practice-guidelines/testosterone-therapy
- **U.S. Anti-Doping Agency – Supplement 411:** https://www.supplement411.org

✨ **Bottom Line for MSM:** If you truly have low testosterone, TRT can change your life — but only when done safely, under medical supervision, and in ways that mimic natural rhythms. Anabolic steroids, HGH, Sermorelin, and shady supplements promise fast gains, but often leave permanent scars on your health. If you choose to use anyway, harm reduction and medical monitoring can help you stay safer.

📊 Gym Supplements & Steroids at a Glance

What Works, What's Hype, What's Harmful
(Remember: Even "safe" supplements can interact with prescription meds or recreational drugs.)

Category	Examples	Evidence & Effectiveness	Cautions / Risks
✅ **Well-Supported / Generally Safe**	**Creatine**	Best evidence for strength & muscle gain.	Avoid with kidney disease; can cause bloating.

Category	Examples	Evidence & Effectiveness	Cautions / Risks
	Whey / Plant Protein Powders	Effective to meet protein needs if diet is lacking.	Some brands high in sugar, fillers, or contaminants.
	Vitamin D	Supports bone, hormone & immune health.	Toxic at high doses.
	Fish Oil (Omega-3s)	May reduce inflammation & support heart health.	Blood-thinning effect.
	Caffeine (coffee, tea, some pre-workouts)	Enhances performance & alertness.	Anxiety, insomnia, blood pressure spikes.
⚖️ Moderate / Limited Evidence	**HMB (β-Hydroxy β-Methylbutyrate)**	May reduce muscle breakdown in beginners/elderly. Less benefit for experienced lifters.	Generally safe, mild GI upset.
	BCAAs (Branched-Chain Amino Acids)	May reduce fatigue during workouts;	Expensive "hype" if diet

Category	Examples	Evidence & Effectiveness	Cautions / Risks
		little added benefit if protein intake adequate.	already has protein.
	Glutamine	Some immune/gut health benefit; little effect on muscle gain.	Harmless but often unnecessary.
	Arginine / Citrulline (NO boosters)	May improve blood flow/pump during workouts.	GI upset, headache; long-term effects unclear.
	DHEA (Dehydroepiandrosterone)	Hormone precursor; mild effect on strength/energy in some studies.	Can alter hormones, acne, mood changes, long-term risks unknown.
	Tribulus terrestris	Marketed as a testosterone booster; human studies show little to no effect.	Often contaminated with undeclared substances.
	Sermorelin (peptide "growth hormone	Not FDA-approved;	Unregulated, purity

Category	Examples	Evidence & Effectiveness	Cautions / Risks
	secretagogue" sold online)	marketed to boost growth hormone.	uncertain, potential for insulin resistance & joint pain.
✕ Risky / Poorly Regulated	**Kratom**	Claimed natural energy/mood booster.	Linked to liver injury, seizures, addiction.
	SARMs (Selective Androgen Receptor Modulators)	Marketed as "legal steroids."	Unregulated, liver toxic, hormonal disruption.
	"Prohormones" (sold OTC)	Steroid precursors, often mislabeled.	Can damage liver, alter hormones.
	High-dose Yohimbine	Promoted for fat burning & libido.	Dangerous spikes in blood pressure, anxiety, heart palpitations.
☠️ Outright Dangerou	**DNP (2,4-Dinitrophenol)**	Used as "fat burner."	Highly toxic; causes fatal

Category	Examples	Evidence & Effectiveness	Cautions / Risks
s / Banned			overheating.
	Clenbuterol (illegal in U.S.)	Beta-agonist used by bodybuilders.	Heart arrhythmias, sudden death risk.
	Anabolic Steroids (non-medical use)	Rapid muscle gain.	Heart disease, infertility, liver damage, mood instability.
	DNTP (designer analogs of DNP sometimes sold online)	Marketed under slightly altered names.	Equally or more toxic than DNP, completely unsafe.

⚠️ **Bottom Line**:

- **Some supplements (creatine, protein, vitamin D) are safe and effective.**
- **Many (Tribulus, "test boosters," BCAAs) are mostly hype.**
- **Some (Kratom, SARMs, DNP/DNTP) are outright dangerous.**
- Even safe supplements can cause **unexpected interactions** with prescription meds or recreational drug

Chapter 19. Ink, Piercings & Cosmetic Procedures – Healing Right and Avoiding Infection

One of my hottest memories as a young gay man took place at a Gold's Gym on the South Shore of Boston. After a workout, I stepped into the gang showers and was joined by an all-American looking guy—broad shoulders, massive quads, the picture of strength. On his back was a giant cross tattoo, and between his legs, a gleaming Prince Albert piercing. He showered next to me, became visibly interested, and later followed me into the sauna. We eventually dated, and like many fantasies, the reality didn't match the dream—he turned out to be a manipulative liar. But the image stayed with me: the raw sexuality of ink and steel, the way tattoos and piercings can transform the body into something tribal, primal, and undeniably hot.

Let's face it—when done tastefully, tattoos, piercings, and even cosmetic enhancements can be incredibly sexy. They're a form of self-expression, a signal of identity, and sometimes a badge of belonging. In the gay community especially, body art can feel like both rebellion and celebration. But along with the allure comes risk. Every needle puncture carries a chance of infection. Poor aftercare, contaminated ink, or an untrained piercer can turn something beautiful into a painful, even dangerous, medical problem.

That's why this chapter exists. We'll dive into how tattoos and piercings affect the body, what can go wrong if they're not done safely, and how to spot and prevent infections. We'll also touch on cosmetic procedures—from fillers to implants—that are increasingly popular among men. The goal isn't to kill the vibe of ink and steel, but to make sure you can enjoy them for what they are: sexy, personal, and safe.

Tattoos, piercings, and cosmetic procedures are highly visible ways MSM express identity, belonging, or sexuality — from a rainbow tattoo to a Prince Albert piercing. But each of these involves breaking the skin or mucosa, which introduces infection risk. In communities already disproportionately impacted by HIV and Hepatitis C, extra care and vigilance are essential.

Tattoos: What to Know Before You Ink

Questions to Ask a Tattoo Artist

- **What ink brands do you use?** Only sterile, regulated, cosmetic-grade inks should be used. Avoid "homemade" or unbranded ink.
- **How do you sterilize equipment?** Autoclaves (steam sterilizers) are gold standard. Avoid any studio without one.
- **Do you use fresh, single-use ink cups and needles?** The answer must be "yes."
- **Do you provide aftercare instructions in writing?** This is a sign of professionalism.

Safer Tattoo Ink Brands

Some tattoo ink brands are known for transparency, sterile manufacturing, and compliance with U.S. and EU safety standards:

- **Eternal Ink** – made in the U.S., vegan-friendly, EU REACH compliant.
- **Intenze Ink** – one of the first FDA-compliant ink companies, sterilized and tested.
- **Dynamic Color Co.** – U.S.-made, high-purity pigments.

- **Fusion Ink** – organic pigments, batch-tested.
- **World Famous Tattoo Ink** – REACH compliant in Europe, transparent labeling.

⚠️ **Avoid:**

- Homemade or "stick-and-poke" inks.
- Black inks with high iron oxide (MRI heating risk).
- Unbranded inks sold online (counterfeits are common).

📌 **Callout Box: Red Flag Tattoo Shops – Walk Out If You See This**

- No autoclave on-site (or unwilling to show you one).
- Reusing ink cups or bottles between clients.
- No gloves or handwashing between customers.
- No visible ink brand labeling or batch codes.
- Refusal to discuss aftercare or dismissing safety questions.

Risks of Tattooing

- **Hepatitis C, HIV, and other bloodborne infections** from contaminated needles or ink.
- **Skin infections** including staph or MRSA.
- **Allergic reactions** (red/yellow inks most common).
- **MRI issues** (iron oxide pigments may heat up).

Piercings & Body Mods

Common Piercing Risks by Location

- **Ear cartilage:** Risk of deforming infection (perichondritis).
- **Navel:** Snagging and very slow healing.
- **Tongue/Lip:** High oral bacteria load → infection risk, chipped teeth.
- **Nipple:** May ooze for weeks, risk of abscess.
- **Genital piercings:** Longer healing times, increased STI risk if condoms break.

Body Modifications

Implants, branding, or scarification often occur outside regulated medical settings. Risks include chronic infections, keloid scarring, and transmission of Hep B, Hep C, or HIV.

Cosmetic Procedures: Fillers, Botox & Beyond

Botox and Other Neurotoxins

Botulinum toxin products reduce wrinkles by relaxing muscles.

- **Botox® (onabotulinumtoxinA):** Gold standard, widely used.
- **Dysport® (abobotulinumtoxinA):** Spreads more easily — useful for larger areas.
- **Xeomin® (incobotulinumtoxinA):** "Naked" form, no accessory proteins — may help in patients who develop resistance.
- **Jeuveau® ("Newtox"):** Marketed to younger patients, slightly lower cost.

⚠️ **Risks:** If improperly injected → drooping eyelids, asymmetric smile, swallowing difficulty. Counterfeit Botox is dangerous and can cause systemic botulism.

Dermal Fillers

Fillers add or restore volume to face, lips, or jawline.

Types of Fillers:

- **Hyaluronic Acid (HA)** – reversible with hyaluronidase.
    - *Brands:* Juvederm®, Restylane®, Belotero®.
    - *Duration:* 6–18 months.
    - *Best for:* Lips, folds, under-eyes.
- **Calcium Hydroxylapatite (CaHA)** – collagen stimulator.
    - *Brand:* Radiesse®.
    - *Duration:* 12–18 months.
    - *Best for:* Jawline, deeper wrinkles.
- **Poly-L-lactic Acid (PLLA)** – builds collagen over time.
    - *Brand:* Sculptra®.
    - *Duration:* 2+ years (several treatments).
    - *Best for:* Facial wasting in HIV, overall volume loss.
- **Polymethylmethacrylate (PMMA)** – semi-permanent.
    - *Brand:* Bellafill®.
    - *Duration:* 5+ years.
    - *Best for:* Deep acne scars, long-term correction.

⚠️ **Risks:**

- **Vascular occlusion** → necrosis, blindness, stroke.
- **Migration or lumps.**
- **Granulomas** (especially with PMMA or silicone).

Botox vs. Fillers

Feature	Botox (Neurotoxin)	Dermal Fillers
Action	Muscle relaxation	Adds/restores volume
Brands	Botox®, Dysport®, Xeomin®, Jeuveau®	Juvederm®, Restylane®, Radiesse®, Sculptra®
Duration	3–6 months	6 months–5+ years
Reversible?	No	HA fillers yes; others no
Main Risks	Drooping, asymmetry, counterfeit dangers	Vascular occlusion, lumps, granulomas

Vetting Your Practitioner

- **Ask which brands are used.** Only FDA-approved products.
- **Demand packaging be opened in front of you.**
- **Verify training/licensure.** Dermatologists, plastic surgeons, or trained NP/PAs.
- **Avoid "Botox parties."** Unsafe, rushed, often with counterfeit drugs.

📌 **Note for MSM with HIV:** Fillers like **Sculptra®** are FDA-approved for HIV-associated lipoatrophy (facial wasting). Insurance may cover it if medically documented.

Healing Right: Aftercare Basics

- Wash hands before touching treated area.
- Gently cleanse with fragrance-free soap.
- Use ointments sparingly.
- Avoid pools, hot tubs, and saunas until healed.
- Do not twist or "spin" fresh jewelry.

Know When to Call a Doctor

- Increasing redness, swelling, or pain
- Pus or foul odor
- Fever or chills
- Allergic reactions (hives, difficulty breathing)
- Persistent bleeding or worsening discharge

What to Ask For if Your Doctor Isn't Familiar

- "Can you culture this?" (for resistant bacteria like MRSA)
- "Can you test me for Hep B, Hep C, HIV?"
- "Should I remove the jewelry, or keep it in for drainage?"
- "Can you refer me to derm or ID if needed?"

📌 **Emergency Red Flags — Call 911 or Go to ER**

- Severe swelling of lip/tongue piercings affecting breathing
- Vision loss or change after filler injection
- Chest pain or shortness of breath after cosmetic injection
- Rapidly spreading redness with fever/chills

Takeaway

Self-expression through ink, piercings, and cosmetic work can be affirming — but only if done safely, with informed choices, and the right aftercare. Know your practitioner, demand transparency, and never be afraid to advocate for your health.

Chapter 20. Mental Health Matters – Depression, Anxiety & Finding LGBTQ-Affirming Help

Back in the early 2000s, when I was still fairly new to practice, I traveled to Saint Louis to visit a friend from Boston. He was one of the friendliest and kindest gay men I knew—handsome, smart, and the kind of guy who could light up a room with his warmth. I had carried a crush on him for years. At the time, he was finishing up his chiropractic program, and we spent hours talking about the future. At one point, he asked me about my experiences with patients struggling with meth addiction. I thought he was speaking academically, as one healthcare student to another. I never suspected he might be speaking from personal pain.

About a year later, I got the devastating news: he had died by suicide. Rumors spread that crystal meth had been part of his struggle, but the truth was never fully shared. What I do know is that depression, addiction, and suicide are deeply intertwined in our community, yet families often silence the story out of shame or misunderstanding. When that happens, the loss remains hidden, and the patterns that lead to tragedy are never fully addressed.

Even today, in Provincetown, we've lost young men to what are delicately called "unexpected deaths." I don't always know the details, but I do know this: when depression, addiction, and suicide are cloaked in secrecy, there is no chance for learning, prevention, or collective healing.

The reality is that depression is epidemic among LGBTQ+ people. Nearly every young gay patient I see is on an SSRI for depression or anxiety. And with today's hostile political climate threatening our safety, rights, and sense of belonging, the burden of mental health challenges in our community is only likely to increase.

This chapter explores depression and anxiety as they uniquely impact LGBTQ+ people, while also highlighting the importance of finding affirming providers—clinicians who understand the cultural context of our struggles and the weight of stigma. Because while the pain is real, so is the possibility of help, healing, and resilience.

Why This Matters for MSM

Mental health is central to overall health, but MSM face unique stressors: stigma, rejection, discrimination, and minority stress. These factors contribute to higher rates of **depression, anxiety, and substance use disorders** compared with the general population. Recognizing symptoms, knowing treatment options, and finding affirming providers can be lifesaving.

Depression in MSM

- **Higher prevalence:** MSM are about **1.5–2×** more likely to experience major depression than heterosexual men.
- **How it can present:** sadness, hopelessness, loss of pleasure; also irritability, fatigue, or changes in sexual interest.
- **Common triggers:** coming out stress, family rejection, internalized homophobia, relationship challenges, body image pressures, HIV stigma/diagnosis.

Evidence-based treatments

- **SSRIs/SNRIs:** effective first-line options (may have sexual side effects—often manageable).
- **Psychotherapy:** Cognitive Behavioral Therapy (CBT) and supportive therapy help reframe negative patterns.
- **Lifestyle support:** exercise, sleep hygiene, social connection.

Anxiety Disorders

- **GAD:** persistent worry, muscle tension, poor sleep.
- **Panic disorder:** sudden episodes of racing heart, breathlessness, chest tightness.
- **Social anxiety:** common after histories of bullying or rejection.

Treatment matters

- **SSRIs** are safest for long-term management.
- **Benzodiazepines** only short-term; long-term use can cause dependence.
- **Therapy** (CBT, mindfulness, acceptance-based approaches) is highly effective.

📌 **Myths vs. Facts – Antidepressants & Therapy**
Myth: "Antidepressants change your personality."
Fact: They reduce symptoms so your real personality can re-emerge.

Myth: "Therapy is only for severe problems."
Fact: It's a tool for stress, relationships, and self-esteem—and many MSM find affirming therapy transformative.

Myth: "SSRIs don't work for gay men."
Fact: They do; responses vary person-to-person. Sometimes pharmacogenomic testing helps.

Myth: "If one med fails, nothing will help."
Fact: There are multiple options and combinations; persistence pays off.

Different Therapy Styles – Finding What Works for You

Not all therapy looks the same. Ask providers which modalities they use and how they adapt them for LGBTQ clients.

- **CBT (Cognitive Behavioral Therapy):** Structured and skills-based; changes unhelpful thoughts/behaviors. Great for depression and anxiety.
- **DBT (Dialectical Behavior Therapy):** CBT + mindfulness + emotion regulation and interpersonal skills; helpful for intense emotions/self-harm urges.
- **Psychodynamic Therapy:** Explores patterns rooted in past experiences; often longer-term for deep self-understanding and relationship themes.
- **ACT/Mindfulness-Based Therapies:** Acceptance and mindfulness to reduce struggle with difficult thoughts/feelings; builds resilience.
- **Group Therapy:** Peer connection in a guided setting; LGBTQ-specific groups can reduce isolation and shame.

- **Couples Therapy (including LGBTQ-affirming models):** Addresses communication, conflict, minority stress in relationships.

☞ **Tip:** If you're unsure, start with CBT or mindfulness-based therapy; add or switch as you learn what fits.

Minority Stress & Internalized Homophobia

Minority stress—stigma, discrimination, concealment—raises depression/anxiety risk.

- **Examples:** hiding relationships at work, microaggressions, family rejection.
- **Internalized homophobia:** shame turned inward.
- **Resilience:** chosen family, LGBTQ community, affirming spirituality.

Suicide Risk

- MSM youth are **~4×** more likely to attempt suicide than heterosexual peers; risk is higher for MSM of color and transgender people.
- **Warning signs:** hopelessness, giving away possessions, increased substance use, sudden calm after distress.

If you or someone you love is thinking of suicide: Call or text **988** (U.S.) or visit **www.988lifeline.org**.

Finding LGBTQ-Affirming Care

Questions to ask

- "How much experience do you have with LGBTQ clients?"
- "How do you address minority stress and intersectionality (race, HIV status, body image)?"
- "What therapy styles do you use, and how are they adapted for LGBTQ folks?"

Where to look

- **GLMA provider directory:** www.glma.org
- **Psychology Today (LGBTQ+ filter):** www.psychologytoday.com
- **National Queer & Trans Therapists of Color Network:** www.nqttcn.com
- **The Trevor Project (youth/young adults):** www.thetrevorproject.org

Practical Tools & Screening

Self-checks to bring to your provider:

- **PHQ-9** (depression)
- **GAD-7** (anxiety)
  Find free versions via **NIMH** (www.nimh.nih.gov) or **APA** (www.psychiatry.org).

When to Contact a Doctor Immediately

- Thoughts of harming yourself or others
- New or worsening panic attacks
- Stopping psychiatric meds abruptly
- **Any seizure** (even if it stops)
- Rapid mood swings or new-onset psychosis

How to Use This Plan

Think of this as your **personal guide**. Start by filling in each section honestly — the more specific you are, the more helpful it will be. Keep a copy somewhere you can easily access (like your phone or wallet), and consider sharing it with a trusted friend, therapist, or partner. Review and update it regularly, especially after changes in your health, medications, or support system. In a crisis, this plan can save time and energy by reminding you — and those helping you — what steps work best for you.

■ My Mental Health Self-Care Plan

This plan is for **me**. It's not a prescription—it's a way to organize what helps me feel grounded, healthy, and safe.

How to Use This Plan

Fill it out honestly and specifically. Keep a copy on your phone/wallet; consider sharing with a trusted friend, partner, or therapist. Revisit it after changes in health, meds, or life stressors. In a crisis, it quickly reminds you—and supporters—what works.

1. My Early Warning Signs

-
-
-

2. My Healthy Coping Tools

- Exercise/movement I enjoy: ______________________________

- Relaxation (meditation, breathwork, prayer): ______________________________

- Creative outlet (music, art, writing): ______________________________

- Social connection (who I reach out to): ______________________________

3. My Support Team

- Friend / chosen family: ______________________________

- Therapist or counselor: ______________________________

- Medical provider: ______________________________

- Crisis support line: ______________________________

4. My Professional Care

- Medications (name & schedule): ______________________________

- Therapy style (CBT, group, mindfulness, etc.): ______________________________

- Screening tools (PHQ-9, GAD-7, etc.): ______________________________

5. My Crisis Plan

- Call **911** for emergencies
- Call/text **988** (Suicide & Crisis Lifeline)

- Local LGBTQ crisis line: ______________________________

- Trusted person to stay with me: ______________________________

6. My Long-Term Goals

-
-
-

☞ **Tip:** Update this plan regularly as your needs change.

Takeaway

Depression and anxiety are **treatable medical conditions**, not personal failings. With an LGBTQ-affirming provider, the right therapy fit, and a practical plan, you can move from surviving to thriving.

Chapter 21. Social Media, Dating Apps & Self-Esteem

I believe social media hasn't just changed us—it's damaged us. Especially for men who have sex with men, the impact has been deeply insidious. Human beings didn't evolve to perceive thousands of potential "suitors" at our fingertips. The illusion of endless choice undermines our ability to focus and commit. There's always someone—just a swipe away—who seems a little better. As a result, commitment becomes elusive. We wear emotional armor, expecting rejection at every turn, even while we may be doing the same to others. The consequence? A persistent tug of insecurity and loneliness, even when we're coupled up.

I don't have a solution—or a way to put the toothpaste back in the tube. But I do know this: relationships today—for my patients and frankly for me—feel shorter, less intimate, and are more fragile. Anxiety and depression are more common than ever. And the data backs this up.

What the numbers say:

- Frequent use of dating apps is linked to **poorer self-esteem**, higher **depression**, and greater **anxiety**—especially when swiping becomes habitual.
- Among MSM, dating app use is associated with increased **body dissatisfaction**, reduced self-esteem, and more mental health strain.
- Young adults who spend more time on social media—regardless of the platform—are **2–3 times more likely** to report feelings of social isolation, depression, and anxiety.

This chapter isn't a moral crusade—it's a recognition. Social media and dating apps were meant to connect us, but their architecture often encourages us to look again, to doubt, to doubt ourselves... to repeat the cycle until we're exhausted.

I may not know how to undo this, but I wrote this chapter because we need to start talking about it. Awareness is the first step toward healing—toward reclaiming focus, presence, and real connection.

Why This Matters for MSM

Social media and dating apps connect MSM to community, friendship, and partners—but they can also amplify body comparison, rejection, compulsive use, and risk behaviors. MSM already experience higher rates of depression than the general male population, which makes understanding these digital effects even more important.

The Upsides

- **Connection & access.** A large share of MSM meet partners online; apps can be a lifeline in less-accepting areas and can even be used to deliver sexual-health info and promote PrEP/testing.

- **Health features are improving.** Audits of MSM-focused apps show increasing (if uneven) integration of HIV-related features, such as PrEP/TasP information and testing prompts.

The Downsides (What Studies Show)

Body Image & Mood

- **Body image pressure via apps.** Qualitative and survey work on Grindr finds body image is shaped by **weight stigma, sexual objectification, and social comparison** unique to the app environment.

- **Higher baseline depression in MSM.** Meta-analysis: depression is **~3×** more prevalent in MSM than in the general male population—so comparison and rejection can hit harder.

Sexual Health & STI Risk

- **Higher risk behavior among app users.** In a study of 1,256 MSM, **46%** used Grindr in the past week; Grindr users reported **more partners and more condomless sex**, and were **more likely to test positive** for chlamydia/gonorrhea (8.6% vs 4.7%).

Substance Use & Chemsex

- **Apps and drug use.** Review data show **app-using MSM** report **59–65% higher rates** of cocaine, ecstasy, methamphetamine, and injection-drug use than non-app-using MSM.

- **Chemsex prevalence.** Among MSM at an Amsterdam STI clinic, **17.6%** reported chemsex in the past 6 months; among gay dating-app users, chemsex was even higher (**29.3%**). Chemsex was linked to **higher bacterial STI risk** in HIV-negative MSM.
- **Mental health impact of chemsex.** Systematic/empirical studies associate chemsex with **depression, anxiety, psychological distress**, and other adverse mental-health outcomes.

Balanced note: Some studies also find that app users are **more engaged with prevention** (e.g., testing and PrEP uptake), suggesting apps can be part of the solution when used thoughtfully.

Practical Strategies for Healthier Use

1. **Curate your feed.** Unfollow accounts that trigger comparison; add diverse, body-positive MSM voices. (Research implicates comparison as a key Grindr mechanism.)
2. **Set limits.** Use screen-time caps and scheduled check-ins.
3. **Mindful swiping.** Ask: "Am I seeking connection—or avoiding loneliness/boredom?"
4. **Phone-free windows.** Make meals, workouts, and hangouts screen-free.
5. **One-week detox each month.** Randomized trials (general population) show **a 1-week social-media break** improves **well-being, depression, and anxiety**; multi-week Facebook/Instagram deactivations also improved well-being. We recommend **one week off per month** as a standing practice.

6. **Balance with real life.** Join LGBTQ sports/arts/volunteer groups to diversify validation beyond apps.

When to Step Back

- You feel worse about yourself after scrolling
- Sleep loss from late-night swiping
- Anxiety, irritability, or FOMO when offline
- Increasing risky encounters or sexualized drug use
- Compulsive use despite wanting to cut back

If these show up, try the **one-week detox** and talk with a therapist or your clinician.

Talking Points with Your Provider

- "I think social media is hurting my self-esteem—what can I do?"
- "What therapy tools help reduce compulsive app use (CBT, mindfulness, DBT skills)?"
- "How can I use apps more safely while building in-person community?"
- "Can we discuss substance-use risk on apps and harm-reduction strategies if chemsex is part of my life?"

Takeaway

For MSM, apps can be both **a lifeline and a stressor**. Evidence links frequent app use to **greater sexual risk, higher substance use (including chemsex), and body-image pressure**, while also showing opportunities for **testing and PrEP engagement**. Curating feeds, setting limits, and taking **a week off every month** are practical, evidence-supported steps to protect mood, sleep, and self-esteem.

📱 My Social Media Balance Plan

This worksheet is for me. It's not a prescription—it's a way to track how social media and dating apps affect my life and set healthier habits.

1. My Main Apps

- Social media I use most: ________________________________

- Dating apps I use most: ________________________________

2. How These Apps Make Me Feel

After 15–30 minutes on an app, I usually feel…

- Better / worse about my body? ______________________________
- Connected / isolated? ____
- Energized / drained? ____
-

3. Warning Signs for Me

When I notice these, it may be time to take a break:

-
-
-

4. My Detox Plan

- I will take **1 week off per month** from all social media/dating apps.

- My next detox week starts: ______________________
- During detox week, I'll spend time doing:
  - In-person connection: ________________________
  - Movement/exercise: ________________________
  - Creative outlets: ____________________________

5. My Healthy App Habits

- Max time per day (minutes): ____________________
- Hours of the day I'll stay offline: _________________
- Accounts I will unfollow to protect my self-esteem: ______
- Accounts I will add for positivity/diversity: __________

6. My Support Team

If apps start harming my mood or leading to risky behavior, these are people I can check in with:

- Friend/chosen family: _________________________
- Therapist/counselor: _________________________
- Provider/doctor: _____________________________

☞ **Tip:** Keep this worksheet on your phone or print it out. Revisit monthly to check progress and adjust.

22. Pets, Purpose & Finding Joy – Why Community (and Dogs) Boost Wellbeing

In the last chapter, I admitted that I don't know of any clear solution for the depression, anxiety, and loneliness that social media and dating apps seem to fuel. But I do know the best counterbalance I've found: having a dog.

My dog has brought such richness and happiness into my life that it's hard to put into words. They are truly man's best friend. Other than the cruelty of their short lives, dogs offer companionship unlike anything else I know. For so many gay men—especially those who live alone or feel the sting of isolation—I recommend the companionship of a dog.

Why? Because dogs have a way of teaching us what no app, no endless swiping, no artificial connection can. They model unconditional love. They remind us to live in the present. They don't care about our status, our body, or our follower count—they care that we came home. Many of them, in their calm presence, are like little Zen masters, holding secrets about patience, presence, and joy that we would do well to learn.

In this chapter, we'll explore why pets—and especially dogs—can play such a powerful role in boosting wellbeing, strengthening community, and reminding us of the deeper truths about love and belonging.

Why Community Matters

Humans are wired for connection. For gay and bisexual men, community has often meant more than friendship—it has been a lifeline. In times of crisis, whether during the early

HIV/AIDS epidemic or more recently during the COVID-19 pandemic, LGBTQ+ communities have shown incredible resilience. Shared meals, chosen family, support groups, Pride events, and even casual neighborhood connections all help buffer against depression, anxiety, and loneliness.

And the science backs this up:

- A meta-analysis of over 300,000 people found that **strong social ties increase survival odds by 50%**—an effect size comparable to quitting smoking (Holt-Lunstad et al., *PLoS Medicine*, 2010).
- Conversely, chronic loneliness increases stress hormones like cortisol, which can raise blood pressure, weaken immunity, and worsen sleep.

For MSM, community connection reduces minority stress—the chronic stress of stigma, discrimination, and concealment—that's strongly linked with depression and anxiety. LGBTQ+ social networks, support groups, and chosen family literally act as buffers against this health risk.

Pets as Partners in Health

Pets—especially dogs—play a unique role in building joy, structure, and connection.

- Pet ownership is booming: as of 2025, **94 million U.S. households**—about **71%**—own at least one pet, up from 82 million in 2023 (Axios; Pet Food Industry).
- Dogs remain the most popular: approximately **51% of households (68 million)** have a dog, while **37% (49 million)** have a cat (American Pet Products Association).

- The American Veterinary Medical Association reports that about **45.5% of households own dogs** and **32.1% own cats** (AVMA).

When it comes to LGBTQ+ populations:

- LGBTQ+ adults are **more likely to be pet parents**, with over **70% of LGBTQ+ adults owning pets compared to 60% of heterosexual adults** (J Lloyd).
- A survey of queer pet parents shows:
    - **89%** turn to pets for comfort,
    - **89%** say pets give them a sense of purpose,
    - **67%** say pets helped them through discrimination,
    - **52%** feel closer to their pets than to family members (Pink News).

Other health benefits are equally well documented:

- The **American Heart Association** has linked dog ownership with **lower cardiovascular risk** and higher physical activity. Dog owners are 34% more likely to meet the recommended 150 minutes of weekly exercise.
- Petting a dog for as little as 5 minutes has been shown to **lower cortisol and increase oxytocin**, improving mood and reducing stress.
- Dog walkers consistently report **higher daily step counts and lower BMI** compared to non-dog owners.

For MSM who may experience isolation, a pet's presence can be grounding. Dogs in particular create opportunities for meeting new people at parks, on walks, or in dog-friendly spaces, while also anchoring daily routines through feeding, walking, and grooming.

Tip: If you've ever felt your mood lift just by coming home to a wagging tail, you've already experienced this effect.

Purpose Beyond Ourselves

Another crucial component of wellbeing is having purpose—something larger than yourself that gives your life meaning.

Research from the **Harvard Study of Adult Development**, the longest-running study of human health, shows that purpose and relationships are the two strongest predictors of long-term wellbeing and happiness.

Purpose might come from:

- Caring for a pet
- Volunteering in LGBTQ+ organizations or broader community service
- Mentoring younger queer men
- Creative work or activism
- Building and sustaining chosen family

Having a sense of purpose has been linked with a **30% lower risk of cognitive decline and depression** in later life.

Finding Joy in Everyday Life

Wellbeing isn't just about avoiding illness; it's about cultivating joy. Consider incorporating:

- **Gratitude journaling:** Multiple randomized trials show it reduces depressive symptoms and improves sleep.
- **Mindful walks:** Pair exercise with stress reduction. Dog walkers in studies report **significantly higher daily step counts** than non-walkers.
- **Play:** Play triggers dopamine release, reducing stress and boosting resilience.
- **Community rituals:** Queer book clubs, sports leagues, volunteer collectives, or spiritual groups provide structure, belonging, and identity affirmation.

Practical Steps to Build Connection & Joy

1. **No pet?** Volunteer at an animal shelter or offer to walk a friend's dog.
2. **Feeling isolated?** Explore LGBTQ+ meetups, hiking clubs, or even online support groups.
3. **Struggling to find purpose?** Ask yourself, *What cause or community lights me up?* Start small with one commitment.
4. **Joy feels elusive?** Try something new—sometimes joy arrives in exploration, not waiting.

✅ Takeaway

Pets, community, and purpose aren't just "nice to have"—they are **foundational to wellbeing**. With **94 million pet-owning households in the U.S.** and especially high ownership among LGBTQ+ adults, pets are essential partners in resilience, connection, and joy. When combined with chosen family and community, they help MSM live healthier, longer, and more joyful lives.

My Joy & Connection Plan

Use this page to reflect on how pets, purpose, and community can support your health. There are no right or wrong answers—this is about *you.*

1. Pets (Current or Future):

- Do you have a pet? If yes, how does your pet bring you joy or structure?

- If no pet, would you like one in the future, or are there ways to connect with animals (shelter volunteering, dog-sitting, visiting friends with pets)?

2. Purpose:

- What gives your life meaning right now? (Work, relationships, creativity, activism, faith, mentoring, etc.)

- What's one small step you could take to grow this sense of purpose?

3. Community:

- Who are the people you can lean on when things get tough?

- Where can you go to feel connected to other LGBTQ+ folks or supportive allies?

- One community activity I'd like to try (support group, queer sports league, book club, volunteer project):

4. Daily Joy Check-In:

- One small thing that brings me joy each day: ____________________________________

- One way I can make space for play or fun this week: ______________________________

✅ **Reminder:** Pets, purpose, and community are as vital to health as diet and exercise. This plan is meant to help you notice where you're already thriving and where you might add more connection and joy.

23. COVID-19, Flu, Mpox & Measles – What's New, What's the Same, and Your Personal Plan

As I write this in 2025, the U.S. Department of Health and Human Services is being led by a non-scientist who is in the process of crippling the ability of the public health sector to respond quickly and scientifically to emerging infectious disease outbreaks. This is not just bureaucratic reshuffling—it's a dismantling of the very infrastructure that kept us afloat during crises like COVID-19 and Mpox.

History has shown, time and again, that men who have sex with men (MSM) are at higher risk for communicable disease outbreaks—from HIV in the 1980s to Mpox in 2022, to localized hepatitis and meningitis outbreaks that still emerge today. For our community, weakening the public health response doesn't just mean slower press conferences or fewer data dashboards—it means greater vulnerability, more infections, and avoidable deaths.

If these damages to our public health system aren't corrected, I fear the next outbreak in the MSM community will be more problematic than it needs to be. Whether it's the resurgence of a familiar threat like flu or measles, or the arrival of a novel pathogen we haven't yet named, our best protection will come from advocating for ourselves, networking to share reliable information, and staying vigilant.

This chapter looks at where we stand now with COVID-19, influenza, Mpox, and measles—what's new, what remains unchanged, and how you can craft your own personal plan. Because the lesson of the last few years is clear: public health may fail us, but we cannot afford to fail one another.

COVID-19: Where We Are Now

COVID-19 is here to stay, but the landscape looks different than in 2020. The virus continues to evolve, with new variants emerging each year. While these newer strains tend to cause less severe disease in most healthy adults, they remain a real risk for older adults, immunocompromised people, and those with chronic illnesses.

- **Vaccines:** Updated COVID-19 vaccines are released annually, much like the flu shot. Data show they continue to reduce the risk of severe disease, hospitalization, and death, even when not a perfect match for circulating variants (CDC, 2024).
- **Treatment:** Antivirals like *nirmatrelvir/ritonavir* (Paxlovid) remain effective if taken within 5 days of symptom onset.
- **Long COVID:** About **5–10% of people** who get COVID may develop long-term symptoms, ranging from fatigue and brain fog to shortness of breath (NIH, 2023). Risk is reduced but not eliminated by vaccination.

Influenza: The Old Foe

Seasonal influenza hasn't gone away—it just got overshadowed. For MSM, the risks mirror those for the general population, but vaccination remains essential.

- **Annual Flu Vaccine:** The flu shot reduces hospitalization risk by 40–60% when well matched to circulating strains (CDC, 2024).
- **Timing:** Best taken in early fall (September–October), but later is better than not at all.

- **High-Risk Groups:** Adults over 50, those with HIV, and anyone with chronic lung, heart, or metabolic conditions are at higher risk of severe flu.

Mpox (Formerly Monkeypox)

The 2022–2023 mpox outbreak disproportionately affected MSM communities worldwide. Since then, numbers have declined, but outbreaks still occur.

- **Transmission:** Primarily through close physical contact, especially sexual contact, but also via contaminated materials (bedding, clothing).
- **Vaccination:** The *JYNNEOS* vaccine is safe and effective.
    - One study found it **reduced mpox risk by 86%** in vaccinated MSM compared to unvaccinated peers (MMWR, 2023).
    - Two doses, 28 days apart, provide the best protection.
- **Symptoms:** Rash, lesions (often painful), fever, and swollen lymph nodes. While often self-limited, mpox can be serious in people with weakened immunity.

Measles: A Preventable but Re-Emerging Threat

Measles, once nearly eliminated in the U.S., has returned in recent years due to declining vaccination rates.

- **Transmission:** Measles is one of the most contagious viruses on earth. If one person has measles, up to **90% of nearby non-immune people** will also become infected.

- **Vaccination:** The MMR (measles, mumps, rubella) vaccine is highly effective—**97% protection** after two doses (CDC, 2024).
- **Why it matters now:** In 2024–2025, multiple outbreaks occurred in U.S. cities and Europe, often spreading in unvaccinated communities. Even brief exposure in airports, gyms, or clubs can lead to infection.
- **For MSM:** Men living with HIV may have less robust protection even if previously vaccinated, and anyone unsure of their vaccination history should ask their provider about an antibody titer or a booster dose.

What's New & What's the Same

- **New:**
    - Annual COVID boosters now work like annual flu shots.
    - Mpox vaccine campaigns remain targeted to MSM and people with multiple partners.
    - Measles outbreaks are back, driven by vaccine hesitancy.
    - Long COVID is increasingly recognized as a chronic health concern.
- **Same:**
    - Handwashing, staying home when sick, and mask use in crowded/poorly ventilated spaces still prevent spread.
    - Vaccines remain the single best tool to prevent severe outcomes.
    - Community solidarity—getting vaccinated, sharing accurate info, checking in on each other—matters.

Future Outlook: Living With Viruses

The reality is that we are entering an age of **viral coexistence**, not eradication. COVID, flu, mpox, and measles remind us that global travel, urban density, and uneven vaccine uptake create a constant backdrop for outbreaks.

- **Pandemics are not one-time events**—they are cycles. Scientists expect other zoonotic viruses to spill over into humans in the coming decades.
- **Climate change** alters disease spread: mosquito-borne viruses (like dengue and Zika) are moving northward.
- **Preparedness matters:** The lesson of HIV, COVID, and mpox is that marginalized communities (like MSM) often face outbreaks first. Building strong, stigma-free public health systems is essential.

The future will depend on **resilience, rapid vaccination, scientific innovation, and community solidarity**. The best defense is a population that is both medically prepared and socially connected.

Your Personal Protection Plan

1. **Vaccinations:**
   - Get your annual flu shot.
   - Stay current on COVID-19 boosters.
   - If eligible (MSM, multiple partners, or at risk), complete the 2-dose JYNNEOS mpox vaccine series.
   - Ensure you've had **two MMR doses** or confirm immunity with a blood test.

2. **Testing & Treatment:**
    - Keep COVID tests at home; test if you have symptoms or a known exposure.
    - Seek prompt treatment if positive—Paxlovid works best within 5 days.
    - For flu, antivirals like oseltamivir (Tamiflu) can shorten illness if started early.
3. **Prevention Habits:**
    - Wash hands often.
    - Ventilate indoor spaces.
    - Wear a mask in crowded public spaces during outbreaks.
    - Stay home when sick.
4. **Community Responsibility:**
    - Share accurate, stigma-free information.
    - Remind friends and partners about vaccine clinics.
    - Support those isolating with groceries, check-ins, or connection.

✅ Takeaway

COVID-19, flu, mpox, and measles are reminders that infectious diseases remain part of our world. The good news: vaccines, antivirals, and community support give us powerful tools to protect ourselves and one another. The future will bring new challenges, but also new solutions—and building your personal plan now is an act of both self-care and community care.

My Seasonal Protection Plan

Use this worksheet to plan ahead and keep track of your prevention steps.

1. Vaccines Checklist:

- Flu shot (date received: ____________)
- COVID-19 booster (date received: ____________)
- Mpox (JYNNEOS) 2-dose series (dates: ____________ / ____________)
- MMR (measles) vaccine or titer check (date: ____________)

2. If I Get Sick:

- My provider/clinic for Paxlovid (COVID) or Tamiflu (flu): ________________________
- Nearest urgent care/ER if severe symptoms: ____________________________________
- Who I'll notify if I test positive: ____

3. Prevention Habits:

- One step I'll take to reduce risk this season (masking, handwashing, ventilation, etc.):
  -
- A reminder to stay home and rest if sick:
  -

4. Community Care:

- How I'll support friends/partners during outbreaks (check-ins, grocery drop-offs, sharing info):
    -

✅ **Reminder:** Planning ahead doesn't just protect you—it protects your community. Vaccines, early treatment, and simple prevention steps are the tools that keep us strong together.

24. Your Emergency Health Kit – Key Documents, Meds, and Contacts in One Place

In the last chapter, we looked at how the dismantling of public health infrastructure—at HHS and beyond—puts communities like ours at heightened risk when the next outbreak or epidemic emerges. But infectious disease isn't the only crisis on the horizon. Across the country, we are watching the slow erosion of institutions that once formed the backbone of public safety: the EPA, OSHA, FEMA, even the agencies tasked with reliable weather prediction. What this means, in plain terms, is that the next public health emergency, natural disaster, or climate-driven crisis will likely be met with less support, less coordination, and fewer resources.

For LGBTQ+ people, the risks are compounded. There are already efforts underway to deny us unique and essential services. Even in 2025, I still can't get insurance coverage for hepatitis B vaccine for some of my patients—something that should be universal given our elevated risks. If we can't get coverage for something so basic, it's hard to imagine that systemic support will improve in a crisis. For patients living with HIV, for example, even something as simple as a pharmacy closure can have devastating consequences. Interruptions in access to antiretrovirals aren't just inconvenient; they can threaten health and survival.

That's why emergency preparedness must be personal. If your insurance allows for 90-day supplies of medication, take advantage of that now. Keep essential documents, medication lists, and emergency contacts organized and accessible. Build redundancy into your health planning so that you aren't entirely dependent on government systems that may falter when you need them most.

This chapter lays out the essentials of creating your own emergency health kit—not out of fear, but out of pragmatism. Because the reality is clear: in a time when institutions are weakened, preparedness is power.

Why an Emergency Health Kit Matters

When life is going smoothly, it's easy to assume you'll always have time to gather what you need. But emergencies—whether a sudden illness, an accident, a natural disaster, or even a last-minute trip—rarely give you time to prepare.

Having an **Emergency Health Kit** ready means that if you need care quickly, you (or someone you trust) can grab one bag and have all the essentials at hand. For MSM, this matters even more: knowing your medications, sexual health history, and advance directives are documented helps ensure you get respectful, appropriate care no matter where you are.

What to Include

1. Key Documents (paper & digital copy):

- Photo ID and insurance card
- Medication list with dosages and prescribing providers
- Allergies (especially drug allergies)
- Vaccination record (COVID, flu, mpox, hepatitis, MMR, tetanus, etc.)

- Copies of recent labs (CD4 count, viral load, hepatitis/HIV/STI tests, cholesterol, etc.)
- Advance directives or healthcare proxy paperwork
- Contact info for your primary care provider and any specialists
- If relevant: documentation for PrEP or HIV treatment, disability status, or transplant history

2. Medications & Supplies:

- At least 7–14 days of your prescription meds in labeled bottles (aim for 30 days if insurance allows)
- Over-the-counter essentials:
    - Acetaminophen or ibuprofen
    - Antihistamines (loratadine, diphenhydramine)
    - Antidiarrheal (loperamide)
    - Oral rehydration packets
    - First-aid basics (bandages, antiseptic wipes)
- Sexual health supplies:
    - Condoms & lube
    - DoxyPEP or PrEP (if prescribed)
- Glasses/contacts with spare case & solution

3. Food & Water Readiness:

- **30 days of shelf-stable rations:** Canned goods, freeze-dried meals, or high-calorie bars. Rotate stock every 6–12 months.
- **RO (Reverse Osmosis) water purification system:** If you own your home, an RO system with UV-C disinfection provides purified water during boil-water advisories, removes lead from aging public infrastructure as well as forever chemical contamination. For renters, consider portable countertop RO systems.

- **Water storage:** At least **1 gallon per person per day** for drinking and hygiene. A 30-day supply = ~30 gallons per person (or store more if space allows).

4. Technology & Backups:

- Portable phone charger / power bank
- Flash drive or cloud folder with all documents scanned
- Battery-powered radio or solar charger
- Extra set of house/car keys

5. Emergency Cash & Contacts:

- Small amount of cash ($50–$100)
- Written list of emergency contacts (friends, family, chosen family, providers) in case your phone dies

6. Pets (because they're family too):

- 7–14 days (ideally 30 days) of pet food
- Any prescription meds your pet takes
- Copies of vaccination records and microchip number
- Extra leash, collar, and ID tags
- Comfort items (blanket, toy) to reduce stress during evacuation
- Portable water/food bowls

MSM-Specific Considerations

- **PrEP/HIV meds:** Even a brief interruption can impact effectiveness. If you're on daily PrEP or HIV therapy, your kit should always have at least a week's supply, preferably 30 days.

- **Stigma in emergencies:** Having medications and documentation labeled reduces awkward or judgmental questions in crisis settings.
- **Community support:** Think beyond yourself—many MSM live alone. A kit means you're more able to assist a friend, partner, neighbor, *or their pets* if disaster strikes.

Sidebar: Emergency Prep for Travelers & Circuit Weekends

Festivals, cruises, and circuit weekends are exciting—but they're also settings where health issues can catch you off guard. A **mini-version of your health kit** is smart travel insurance.

Pack for every trip:

- 3–5 days of your daily prescription meds in original bottles
- Small pill organizer with OTC basics (pain reliever, antacid, antihistamine, loperamide)
- A few oral rehydration packets (great after partying or if you get food poisoning)
- Condoms, lube, and DoxyPEP/PrEP (if prescribed)
- Copy of your vaccine record and provider contact info in your phone
- Portable phone charger and backup power bank
- $50 cash (not every bar/club/festival booth takes cards)

Why this matters:

- Long weekends often mean **strained local clinics** and long waits at urgent cares.
- In places with stigma or language barriers, having your meds and records avoids delays.
- If your phone is lost or dies, a small paper backup of your provider and emergency contact numbers is invaluable.

Tip: Treat your travel kit as "carry-on only." Always keep meds and key documents in your carry-on bag—not checked luggage.

Keeping It Updated

- **Check every 6 months:** Replace expired meds, rotate food/water, refresh pet supplies, and update documents.
- **Digital + physical:** Keep a copy in your phone's health app or cloud storage *and* in a physical folder.
- **Trusted person:** Tell someone you trust where your kit is stored.

✅ Takeaway

Emergencies happen fast—but a little preparation makes them far less stressful. Whether it's a trip to the ER, a hurricane knocking out power and water, or a long weekend away, your **Emergency Health Kit** ensures you always have what you need. For some, a 7–14 day kit is enough; for others, aiming for **30 days of supplies, food, water, and pet care** is the ultimate peace of mind.

My Emergency Health Kit Checklist

1. Documents

- Photo ID & insurance card
- Medication list & allergies
- Vaccination record
- Recent labs
- Advance directive/healthcare proxy
- Provider contact info
- HIV/PrEP treatment documentation

2. Medications & Supplies

- 7–30 day supply of prescriptions or up to 90 days if your insurance plan will allow
- Pain reliever (acetaminophen/ibuprofen)
- Antihistamine
- Antidiarrheal
- Oral rehydration packets
- First-aid basics
- Condoms & lube
- DoxyPEP or PrEP (if prescribed)
- Glasses/contacts

3. Food & Water

- 30 days of shelf-stable food
- 1 gallon of water per person per day (minimum)
- Reverse Osmosis system or water filter

4. Tech & Backups

- Portable phone charger / solar charger
- Flash drive or cloud backup of documents
- Battery-powered radio
- Extra house/car keys

5. Cash & Contacts

- $50–$100 cash
- Written list of emergency contacts

6. Pets

- 7–30 days of pet food
- Pet medications
- Vaccination records & microchip number
- Leash/collar with ID tags
- Comfort items (blanket, toy)
- Portable bowls

Maintenance Plan:

- Next update due: ______________________
- Person who knows where my kit is: ______________________

✅ **Reminder:** Caring for yourself also means caring for the beings who rely on you—whether that's a partner, chosen family, or a pet. Build your kit once, and you'll thank yourself when you need it.

Appendix A – Doctor Visit Checklist

Why a Checklist Matters

Doctor visits can feel rushed, especially in busy practices. It's common to leave the office only to remember the one question you *really* wanted answered. A **Doctor Visit Checklist** helps you make the most of your time, ensures you don't forget important concerns, and gives your provider a clear picture of your health.

For MSM, a checklist is even more valuable—sexual health, mental health, substance use, and preventive care needs may not always be asked about unless you bring them up. This tool makes sure nothing slips through the cracks.

Before Your Visit

- **Update your medication list** (prescriptions, PrEP, HIV meds, over-the-counter, supplements).
- **Track your symptoms**: When they started, how often they happen, what makes them better or worse.
- **Check your vaccinations**: COVID booster, flu shot, mpox, hepatitis A/B, HPV, MMR, tetanus.
- **Review your sexual health needs**: STI testing, PrEP follow-up, DoxyPEP refills, HIV care.
- **List your top 2–3 priorities** for this visit. (Example: "Discuss fatigue," "Check cholesterol," "Ask about anxiety.")

During Your Visit

- **Bring your written list of questions** so you don't forget.
- **Share your mental health status** (depression, anxiety, stress, substance use).
- **Be honest about sexual health**—partners, practices, condom/DoxyPEP use. Your provider can only help with what they know.
- **Ask about labs and follow-ups**: When, how, and who will contact you with results.
- **Request explanations in plain language** if something isn't clear.

After Your Visit

- **Review your visit summary** (often available via patient portal).
- **Schedule any labs, imaging, or referrals** right away so they don't get forgotten.
- **Note medication changes**—dose, frequency, and side effects to watch for.
- **Write down next steps**: When is your next visit? What lifestyle or self-care goals were recommended?

My Doctor Visit Worksheet

Today's Date: ______________________
Provider: __________________________

My Top 3 Priorities:

1.
2.
3.

Medications I'm Taking Now:

-
-
-

Symptoms or Concerns I Want to Discuss:

-
-

Sexual Health Needs:

- STI testing
- PrEP refill or monitoring
- HIV treatment/lab follow-up
- DoxyPEP prescription/refill
- HPV vaccine discussion
- Other: ______________________________

Mental Health Check-In:

- Mood over the past 2 weeks: ______________________________
- Anxiety or stress triggers: ______________________________

Questions for My Doctor:

-
-
-

Next Steps (after visit):

-
-

✅ **Tip:** Print a few copies of this worksheet, keep them in a folder with your medical papers, and fill one out before each appointment. This way, your visits stay focused and you get the care you deserve.

Appendix B – Glossary of Sexual-Health & LGBTQ+ Terms

This glossary is designed to give quick, easy-to-understand explanations of common terms in sexual health, LGBTQ+ identities, and community culture. Language evolves, and people use words differently based on culture, generation, and identity. When in doubt, ask someone what words they use for themselves and their body.

A

Ace (Asexual): Someone who experiences little or no sexual attraction. Some still have sex or relationships, others do not.

Agender: A person who does not identify with any gender.

Anal Douching (Enema): Flushing the rectum with water or saline before sex to feel clean. Best done with isotonic solutions to avoid irritation.

Anal Sex: Penetration of the anus with a penis, finger, or sex toy. Also called "bottoming" for the receptive partner and "topping" for the insertive partner.

Aromantic (Aro): Someone who experiences little or no romantic attraction to others.

B

Barebacking: Condomless anal sex. Sometimes intentional, sometimes spontaneous. Carries risks for HIV and other STIs.

Bear: A gay man, often larger and hairier, who embodies a rugged or masculine aesthetic. Associated with its own subculture.

Bottom: A person who takes the receptive role in anal sex. (See also: Top, Versatile.)

Buddy/Chosen Family: Non-biological friends who provide support, care, and love, often standing in where biological family may not.

Bump: Slang for a small inhaled dose of a powdered drug (often cocaine, ketamine, or meth).

C

Chemsex: Using drugs (such as meth, GHB, mephedrone, ketamine, cocaine) to enhance or prolong sex. Can increase risks of STI transmission, addiction, and overdose.

Cisgender: A person whose gender identity matches the sex they were assigned at birth.

Coming Out: The process of sharing your LGBTQ+ identity with others. May happen many times in different contexts.

Consent: Clear, informed, and voluntary agreement to participate in sexual activity. Can be withdrawn at any time.

Crystal / Tina / Ice: Slang terms for methamphetamine, a powerful stimulant often linked to chemsex and high addiction risk.

Cruising: Seeking anonymous or casual sexual encounters, often in public or semi-public spaces.

Circuit Party: A large dance event in LGBTQ+ culture, often involving electronic music, costumes, and sometimes sexual expression and drug use.

Coke / Snow: Slang for cocaine, a stimulant drug often snorted or rubbed on gums.

D

DoxyPEP: Taking doxycycline (an antibiotic) within 72 hours after sex to reduce risk of syphilis, chlamydia, and sometimes gonorrhea.

Down Low (DL): A term sometimes used for men who have sex with men but do not identify as gay or bisexual, often keeping it secret.

Drag: Performance art involving exaggerated gender expression, usually through clothing, makeup, and performance.

F

Felching: The act of sucking semen out of someone's anus after anal sex. Risk for STIs if performed without protection.

Fetish: Sexual arousal linked to a specific object, body part, or activity. Can be part of healthy sexual expression when practiced consensually.

Fisting: Insertion of a whole hand into the rectum or vagina, requiring preparation, communication, and safety practices.

420: Slang for cannabis (marijuana). Commonly used to signal interest in smoking or using weed.

G

Gay: A person (usually a man) who is romantically or sexually attracted to other men.

Gender Identity: A person's internal sense of being male, female, both, neither, or another gender.

Gender Expression: The way a person presents themselves outwardly (clothing, hairstyle, behavior), which may or may not align with societal expectations.

Gender Dysphoria: Distress that occurs when someone's gender identity does not match their sex assigned at birth.

Grindr (or Dating Apps): A popular app among MSM for meeting sexual or romantic partners.

G (GHB): Slang for gamma-hydroxybutyrate, a sedative drug used recreationally in chemsex. Overdose risk is high due to narrow dosing window.

H

HIV (Human Immunodeficiency Virus): The virus that, if untreated, can lead to AIDS. Managed today with effective antiretroviral therapy.

Hookup: Casual sexual encounter, often arranged via apps, clubs, or events.

HPV (Human Papillomavirus): A common sexually transmitted virus that can cause warts or cancers. Preventable with vaccination.

K

Kink: Sexual practices outside mainstream norms that focus on power, sensation, or role play. Examples: bondage, dominance/submission, impact play. Healthy when consensual, safe, and respectful.

K (Ketamine / "Special K"): A dissociative anesthetic used recreationally for its hallucinogenic and numbing effects. Common in club and chemsex scenes.

L

Lesbian: A woman who is romantically or sexually attracted to women.

Lube (Lubricant): A substance that reduces friction during sex. Water-based is condom safe; silicone lasts longer; avoid oil with latex condoms.

M

MSM (Men Who Have Sex with Men): Public health term describing behavior, not identity.

Mpox (Monkeypox / MPX): A viral infection spread by close contact or sex. Preventable with the JYNNEOS vaccine.

Molly / E / X: Slang for MDMA (ecstasy), a stimulant and empathogen often used in clubs or raves.

N

Nonbinary: Someone whose gender identity does not fit within the male/female binary.

NAAT (Nucleic Acid Amplification Test): A sensitive lab test used for detecting STIs like gonorrhea, chlamydia, and *Mycoplasma genitalium.*

P

PrEP (Pre-Exposure Prophylaxis): HIV prevention medicine (pills or injections) taken before exposure.

PEP (Post-Exposure Prophylaxis): HIV medicine taken within 72 hours after potential exposure.

Party and Play (PnP): Using drugs (commonly meth, G, K) during sex. Often overlaps with chemsex.

Pansexual: Someone who can be attracted to people regardless of gender.

R

Rimming: Oral stimulation of the anus. Risk for STIs like gonorrhea, chlamydia, HPV, and hepatitis A.

S

Snowballing: The act of kissing and passing semen from one mouth to another.

Shrimping: Sucking on another person's toes.

Stealthing: Non-consensual removal of a condom during sex. Considered sexual assault in many jurisdictions.

Switch: Someone who enjoys both dominant and submissive roles in kink or BDSM.

T

Top: A person who takes the insertive role in anal sex.

Tina: Slang for methamphetamine (see also Crystal, Ice).

Transgender: Someone whose gender identity is different from the sex they were assigned at birth.

Twink: A gay man, usually young, slim, little body hair, often associated with a boyish look.

U–W

U=U (Undetectable = Untransmittable): People with HIV on ART and an undetectable viral load cannot transmit HIV sexually.

Versatile (Vers / Switch): Someone who enjoys both topping and bottoming in sex.

WLW (Women Loving Women): Inclusive term for women attracted to women.

Clinical Acronyms & Abbreviations Cheat Sheet

Abbreviation	Meaning	Why It Matters
HIV	Human Immunodeficiency Virus	Virus that attacks the immune system; prevented with PrEP, treated with ART.
ART	Antiretroviral Therapy	Daily HIV meds that keep virus suppressed; basis of U=U.
PrEP	Pre-Exposure Prophylaxis	HIV prevention pills or injections.
PEP	Post-Exposure Prophylaxis	HIV meds taken within 72 hours after possible exposure.
MSM	Men Who Have Sex with Men	Behavior-based public health term.
WLW	Women Loving Women	Inclusive term for women attracted to women.
HCV	Hepatitis C Virus	Bloodborne liver infection, curable with antivirals.
HBV	Hepatitis B Virus	Liver infection spread by sex, blood, or birth. Vaccine-preventable.
HBsAg	Hepatitis B Surface Antigen	Lab marker showing active HBV infection.
HPV	Human Papillomavirus	STI causing genital warts and cancers.
E6/E7	HPV Oncoproteins	Linked to cancer development.

Abbreviation	Meaning	Why It Matters
MG	*Mycoplasma genitalium*	Bacterial STI, harder to treat.
GC	*Neisseria gonorrhoeae*	Bacterium that causes gonorrhea.
CT	*Chlamydia trachomatis*	Bacterium that causes chlamydia.
NAAT	Nucleic Acid Amplification Test	DNA-based lab test for STIs.
MPX	Mpox (Monkeypox)	Viral infection spread by close contact.
HRT	Hormone Replacement Therapy	Used in gender-affirming care.

📑 Lab-Slip Decoder – Understanding Your STI & Viral Test Results

Lab Test Code	Plain Language	What It Means
HIV Ag/Ab (4th Gen)	HIV antigen/antibody combo test	Detects both virus and immune response; picks up HIV earlier.
RPR / VDRL	Syphilis screening	Antibody blood test; positives need

Lab Test Code	Plain Language	What It Means
		confirmatory testing.
NAAT (GC, CT, MG)	DNA-based test	Detects gonorrhea, chlamydia, and *Mycoplasma genitalium*.
GC	*Neisseria gonorrhoeae*	Bacterium causing gonorrhea.
CT	*Chlamydia trachomatis*	Bacterium causing chlamydia.
MG	*Mycoplasma genitalium*	STI that can cause persistent urethritis or proctitis.
HBsAg	Hepatitis B surface antigen	Positive = active infection.
Anti-HBs	Hepatitis B surface antibody	Positive = immunity (from vaccine or past infection).
HCV Ab	Hepatitis C antibody	

Lab Test Code	Plain Language	What It Means
		Positive = past exposure; needs RNA test for active infection.
HPV (E6/E7 mRNA)	HPV activity test	Detects high-risk viral activity linked to cancer.
Mpox PCR	Test for Mpox virus	Detects active Mpox infection.

Appendix C:

Helplines, Hotlines, and Provider Finder Resources for Men Who Have Sex with Men (MSM)

Purpose of This Appendix

Finding affirming, competent, and accessible care can be one of the most powerful steps you take in protecting your health. Whether you're seeking mental health support, HIV prevention or treatment, substance use services, crisis intervention, or LGBTQ+ affirming providers, the following resources are curated to connect you quickly and confidentially with the right support — wherever you are.

1. LGBTQ+ and General Crisis Hotlines

Immediate Crisis or Emotional Support

- **988 Suicide & Crisis Lifeline**
  📞 Dial **988** (24/7, free, confidential)
  □ 988lifeline.org
  For anyone experiencing emotional distress, suicidal thoughts, or substance-related crises. You can also text **988** or use chat online.
- **The Trevor Project (for LGBTQ+ youth and young adults)**
  📞 1-866-488-7386 | Text **START** to 678-678
  □ thetrevorproject.org/get-help
  24/7 crisis intervention and suicide prevention for LGBTQ+ youth up to age 25.
- **Trans Lifeline**
  📞 1-877-565-8860 (U.S.) | 1-877-330-6366 (Canada)
  □ translifeline.org

Peer support for trans and nonbinary individuals by trans and nonbinary operators.

- **LGBT National Help Center**
  📞 1-888-843-4564
  □ lgbthotline.org
  General information, peer support, and referrals for LGBTQ+ adults.
  Also offers:
    - **Youth Talkline:** 1-800-246-PRIDE
    - **Senior Hotline:** 1-888-234-7243

2. HIV, PrEP, and Sexual Health Hotlines

- **CDC National HIV/AIDS Hotline**
  📞 1-800-232-4636 (English & Spanish)
  □ cdc.gov/hiv
  Offers confidential information about HIV testing, prevention, and treatment.
- **HIV.gov Provider & Service Locator**
  □ locator.hiv.gov
  Find nearby PrEP providers, HIV testing sites, PEP access, Ryan White clinics, and other HIV care services.
- **Hepatitis B Foundation Helpline**
  📞 1-215-489-4900
  □ hepb.org
  Expert support and education for individuals living with or at risk for hepatitis B.
- **Hepatitis C Warmline (University of California, San Francisco)**
  📞 1-800-933-3413 | M–F 9AM–8PM ET
  □ nccc.ucsf.edu/clinician-consultation
  Clinician-to-clinician consult line, but can also guide patients toward knowledgeable providers.

- **PrEP Locator (CDC & NASTAD)**
  □ preplocator.org
  Find PrEP-prescribing clinics, telehealth services, and pharmacies in your area.
- **PleasePrEPMe**
  □ pleaseprepme.org
  U.S.-based and international PrEP navigation, including telehealth and insurance support.

3. LGBTQ+ Affirming Provider and Health Center Finders

- **GLMA: Health Professionals Advancing LGBTQ+ Equality**
  □ glma.org → *Find a Provider* directory
  Verified LGBTQ+ affirming healthcare professionals across all specialties.
- **Plume Health**
  □ getplume.co
  Telehealth-based gender-affirming care (hormones, labs, letters, etc.) for adults.
- **FOLX Health**
  □ folxhealth.com
  LGBTQ+ centered telehealth platform for PrEP, HRT, and general wellness.
- **Q Care Plus**
  □ qcareplus.com
  Online PrEP and HIV care services for MSM and LGBTQ+ individuals nationwide.
- **Planned Parenthood LGBTQ+ Services**
  □ plannedparenthood.org
  Offers sexual health, hormone therapy, STI screening, and PrEP/PEP in many locations.
- **CenterLink LGBTQ+ Community Center Directory**
  □ lgbtcenters.org

Find local community health centers and LGBTQ+ organizations near you.

4. Substance Use, Recovery, and Harm Reduction Resources

- **SAMHSA National Helpline**
  📞 1-800-662-HELP (4357) | 24/7, confidential, free
  □ findtreatment.gov
  For substance use or mental health treatment referrals.
- **Never Use Alone Hotline**
  📞 1-800-484-3731
  For people using substances alone — stay on the line with a trained operator for safety monitoring and emergency dispatch if needed.
- **NARCAN Finder (NIDA)**
  □ narcan.com/buy-narcan
  Locate nearby pharmacies or organizations offering free or discounted naloxone.
- **Harm Reduction Coalition**
  □ harmreduction.org
  National directory of harm reduction services, safe syringe access, and overdose prevention programs.
- **Shatterproof Treatment Atlas**
  □ treatmentatlas.org
  Compare addiction treatment programs and recovery options by state.

5. Mental Health and Emotional Wellness

- **National Alliance on Mental Illness (NAMI) Helpline**
  📞 1-800-950-NAMI (6264) | Text "HELPLINE" to

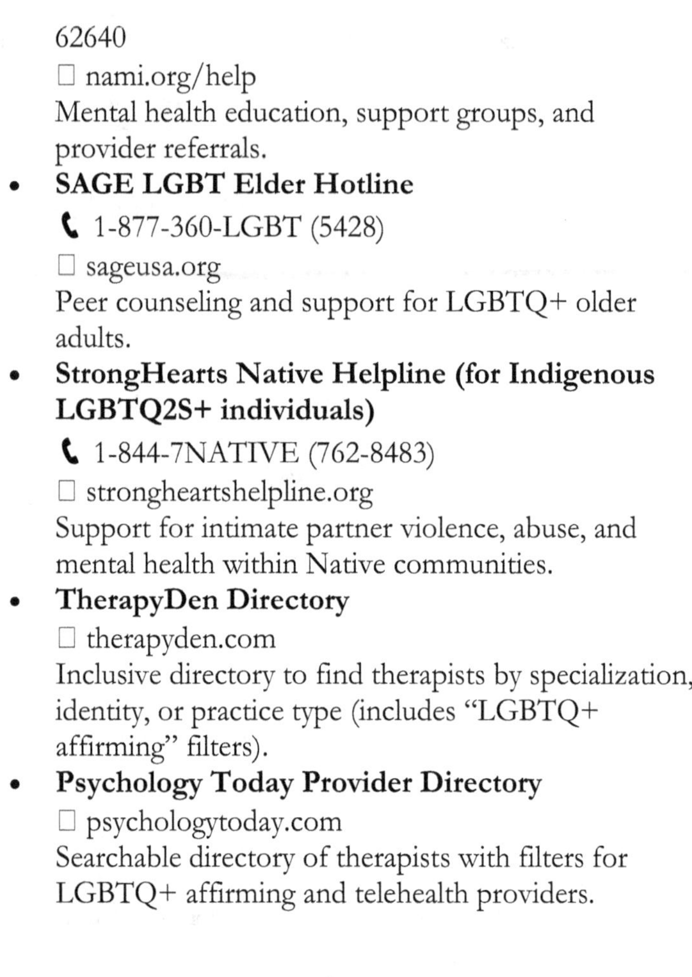

62640
☐ nami.org/help
Mental health education, support groups, and provider referrals.

- **SAGE LGBT Elder Hotline**
  📞 1-877-360-LGBT (5428)
  ☐ sageusa.org
  Peer counseling and support for LGBTQ+ older adults.
- **StrongHearts Native Helpline (for Indigenous LGBTQ2S+ individuals)**
  📞 1-844-7NATIVE (762-8483)
  ☐ strongheartshelpline.org
  Support for intimate partner violence, abuse, and mental health within Native communities.
- **TherapyDen Directory**
  ☐ therapyden.com
  Inclusive directory to find therapists by specialization, identity, or practice type (includes "LGBTQ+ affirming" filters).
- **Psychology Today Provider Directory**
  ☐ psychologytoday.com
  Searchable directory of therapists with filters for LGBTQ+ affirming and telehealth providers.

6. Legal, Discrimination, and Advocacy Support

- **Lambda Legal Help Desk**
  📞 1-866-542-8336
  ☐ lambdalegal.org/helpdesk
  Legal information and assistance for LGBTQ+ individuals facing discrimination in healthcare, employment, or housing.

- **National Center for Transgender Equality (NCTE)**
  □ transequality.org
  Guides on name/gender marker changes, health insurance coverage, and rights in healthcare.
- **Human Rights Campaign Healthcare Equality Index**
  □ hrc.org/hei
  Rates hospitals and clinics based on their LGBTQ+ inclusivity and policies.

7. International and Global Health Resources

- **UNAIDS MSM Health Resources**
  □ unaids.org
  Global data, rights-based information, and service networks for MSM and people living with HIV.
- **ILGA World (International Lesbian, Gay, Bisexual, Trans and Intersex Association)**
  □ ilga.org
  Directory of regional advocacy and support organizations across 170+ countries.
- **Global Black Gay Men Connect**
  □ gbgmc.org
  Global advocacy and support network focused on the health and rights of Black gay and bisexual men.

8. Telehealth, At-Home Testing, and Digital Health Options

- **MISTR**
  □ heymistr.com
  Free online PrEP, telemedicine visits, and lab testing in all 50 states.

- **MyLab Box**
  □ mylabbox.com
  Discreet at-home STI, HIV, and wellness testing kits.
- **Nurx**
  □ nurx.com
  Telehealth prescriptions for PrEP, STI testing, and general sexual health.
- **LetsGetChecked**
  □ letsgetchecked.com
  Home testing for HIV, STIs, hormone levels, and more.

9. In Case of Emergency

If you or someone you know is in **immediate danger or experiencing a medical emergency**, **dial 911** (U.S.) or go to the nearest emergency department.

If you are in crisis but prefer text support:
📱 Text **HOME** to **741741** to reach the **Crisis Text Line**, available 24/7 across the U.S. and Canada.

Final Note

Empowerment comes from access — and access comes from knowing where to turn. Keep this appendix saved, shared, and visible. You deserve informed, compassionate, and affirming care — *always*.

www.ingramcontent.com/pod-product-compliance
Lightning Source LLC
Chambersburg PA
CBHW050701280326
41926CB00088B/2414

9798218832117